Fibro Flare
No More
4-in-1 Fibromyalgia Relief Book

Your Comprehensive Guide & Cookbook
Understand Symptoms, Navigate Treatments, Embrace Life
with Effortless, Quick, Anti-Inflammatory Recipes

Liv Marwin

To Myself, My Family,
and all those silently
battling fibromyalgia:
Your strength inspires.
Your resilience empowers.
This book is for us.

TABLE OF CONTENT

INTRODUCTION

FOREWORD BY THE AUTHOR

Hello, fellow fibromyalgia warriors! Welcome to "Fibro Flare No More: The Ultimate 4-in-1 Fibromyalgia Relief Book". This book is my heartfelt contribution to our shared journey, and I'm here to support and empower you as we navigate this challenging condition together.

I'm right there with you in this struggle. Like many of you, I've spent years dealing with persistent pain and overwhelming fatigue. Receiving a fibromyalgia diagnosis was both a relief and the beginning of a new, complex journey.

This book encompasses everything I wish I had known from the start. It's the result of extensive research, countless conversations with other fibromyalgia patients, and personal experiences - both the successes and the setbacks.

I vividly recall the moment I decided to take control of my health. I realized that managing fibromyalgia isn't just about medication or following a prescribed treatment plan. It's about comprehensively changing our lifestyle. This realization led me to explore various aspects of living with fibromyalgia, including nutrition, symptom management, traditional and holistic treatments, and strategies for daily life.

This book is a complete guide. It covers understanding and managing symptoms, exploring both conventional and alternative treatments, and provides practical advice for living with this condition. While it does include nutritional information and recipes, that's just one part of the comprehensive approach we'll explore.

Let's address something important - the feeling of isolation that often comes with fibromyalgia. It's crucial to remember that we're not alone in this. The stories and testimonials in this book are a testament to our shared experiences and the strength of our community.

I understand that fibromyalgia is not just a physical challenge. It affects our mental and emotional well-being too. Those days when the pain is overwhelming and fatigue makes even simple tasks difficult can take a toll on our mental health. That's why I've included strategies for maintaining emotional wellness alongside physical health.

As you read through these pages, you'll find a mix of practical advice, scientific information (presented in an accessible way), and personal insights. My goal is to provide you with the knowledge and tools you need to effectively manage your symptoms and improve your quality of life.

Thank you for choosing this book. Whether you're newly diagnosed or have been living with fibromyalgia for years, I hope you'll find valuable information and support within these pages. Remember, you have incredible strength within you. With the right tools and support, you can navigate this condition and find a path to better health and well-being.

Wishing you strength and healing, 								*Liv Marwin*

HOW TO USE THIS BOOK

Navigating life with fibromyalgia can be overwhelming, but this book is designed to be your comprehensive guide. Whether you're newly diagnosed or have been living with fibromyalgia for years, this book will offer practical advice, evidence-based strategies, and personal stories to help you manage your symptoms and improve your quality of life. Here's how to get the most out of this resource:

First and foremost, **start with the Table of Contents**. This will give you a clear overview of the book's structure and help you identify the sections that are most relevant to your current needs. The book is divided into four main parts: Understanding Fibromyalgia, Meal Plans and Recipes, Treatments and Symptom Management, and Living with Fibromyalgia. Each part is designed to address different aspects of managing fibromyalgia, from understanding your diagnosis to finding the best treatments and support systems.

Feel free to skip around. While the book is structured to be read from start to finish, it's also meant to be a resource you can dip into as needed. If you're currently struggling with sleep issues, head straight to the chapter on Sleep Hygiene. If you're looking for new recipes to try, explore the Meal Plans and Recipes section. Each chapter is self-contained, providing valuable information and strategies that you can apply immediately.

Use the practical tips and action steps. Each chapter concludes with actionable advice that you can incorporate into your daily life. These tips are designed to be straightforward and easy to implement, helping you make small changes that can lead to significant improvements in your symptoms and overall well-being.

Take advantage of the patient stories and testimonials. These personal accounts are woven throughout the book to provide real-life examples of people who have successfully managed their fibromyalgia. These stories offer hope and inspiration, showing that it is possible to live a fulfilling life despite the challenges of fibromyalgia.

Engage with the interactive features. This book includes various interactive elements such as symptom trackers, progress charts, and QR codes linking to video tutorials. These tools are designed to help you monitor your symptoms, track your progress, and access additional resources that can support your journey.

Keep a journal. Consider using a journal to document your experiences as you work through the strategies in this book. Writing down your thoughts, challenges, and victories can be a powerful tool for reflection and growth. It can also help you identify patterns in your symptoms and responses to different treatments, providing valuable insights for your healthcare providers.

Build your support network. One of the key themes of this book is the importance of community and support. Use the information and resources provided to connect with others who understand what you're going through. Whether it's joining a local support group, participating in online forums, or simply talking to friends and family, building a support network can make a significant difference in your journey with fibromyalgia.

Stay updated. Medical research and treatment options for fibromyalgia are continually evolving. This book provides a solid foundation of current knowledge, but it's essential to stay informed about new developments. Consider subscribing to reputable medical journals, joining fibromyalgia advocacy groups, or setting up news alerts to keep up with the latest research and advancements in treatment.

Finally, **be patient with yourself**. Managing fibromyalgia is a marathon, not a sprint. Progress may be slow, and setbacks are inevitable. Use this book as a steady companion, offering guidance and support through the ups and downs. Celebrate your small victories, and remember that each step forward, no matter how small, is a step towards better health and a better quality of life.

By following these guidelines, you can make the most of this book and take proactive steps towards managing your fibromyalgia.

INTRODUCTION TO FIBROMYALGIA

MY PERSONAL STORY WITH FIBROMYALGIA

When I was first diagnosed with fibromyalgia, it felt like stepping into an entirely new world—one filled with uncertainty and relentless challenges. For two years, I endured inexplicable pain, often fearing I was losing my mind. There were moments when I thought I was imagining everything because the pain would move from one part of my body to another throughout the day, only to vanish and reappear elsewhere. Yet, deep down, I knew something was truly wrong.

Some mornings, I didn't have the strength to get out of bed. Even simple activities felt impossible, forcing me to change my daily routines drastically. Many days, I felt lazy and believed it was just a matter of willpower. The fatigue and pain were overwhelming, making even the simplest tasks feel monumental. Nights were often sleepless, adding to my sense of despair and exhaustion.

The journey to a diagnosis was long and frustrating. Numerous doctor visits and countless tests left me feeling alone and bewildered. Not knowing what was wrong with me made everything worse, and I often questioned my sanity. There were times when I thought I was simply imagining the pain, and the lack of answers made me feel hopeless.

However, this struggle ignited a fire within me—a determination not only to manage my condition but also to help others navigating the same turbulent waters. The day I finally received my diagnosis was a profound relief; at last, I had a name for two years of unexplained pain and suffering. It brought a sense of validation to know that my experience had a cause and that I wasn't alone or imagining my symptoms.

Living with fibromyalgia takes immense courage. The constant battle with pain and fatigue can be disheartening, but I realized that sharing my experiences and the knowledge I accumulated could provide solace and guidance to many. I want others to know that their struggles are real and that it's okay to feel overwhelmed. It's important to seek professional advice and support, and to understand that managing fibromyalgia is a continuous journey.

There were many days when I felt defeated, thinking my lack of energy and constant pain were signs of laziness. But I knew deep down that I wasn't well, and I learned that fibromyalgia is a serious condition that requires understanding, patience, and strength. The fatigue and pain aren't just in our heads; they are real and can significantly impact our lives.

This book is my way of reaching out to you, offering a beacon of hope and a reservoir of practical advice to manage fibromyalgia effectively. I hope that by opening my heart and sharing my journey, I can light a path for those who feel lost in the darkness of this condition. You are not alone, and together, we can find strength, resilience, and hope.

Understanding fibromyalgia and finding ways to cope with it has been a challenging yet enlightening experience. It has taught me the importance of self-care and the need to listen to my body. I've learned to pace myself and to celebrate small victories. Every day is a step forward, and every challenge is an opportunity to grow stronger.

If you are struggling with fibromyalgia, remember that it takes immense courage to face each day. Don't be too hard on yourself and seek support whenever you need it. There is a community of people who understand what you're going through, and together, we can navigate this journey with compassion and strength.

OVERVIEW OF FIBROMYALGIA

Fibromyalgia is a chronic illness marked by widespread musculoskeletal pain, tiredness, and soreness in specific locations. The term "fibromyalgia" comes from "fibro," referring to fibrous tissues, "my," meaning muscle, and "algia," indicating pain. This condition affects millions of people worldwide, predominantly women, and it significantly impacts their quality of life.

Understanding the Symptoms

Widespread pain, which is commonly defined as a persistent dull aching that lasts for at least three months, is the main symptom of fibromyalgia. Usually, the discomfort is experienced above and below the waist, as well as on both sides of the body. In addition to pain, fibromyalgia patients frequently have extreme exhaustion, disturbed sleep patterns, and cognitive impairments, sometimes known as "fibro fog." This cognitive impairment can affect memory, attention, and the ability to concentrate, making daily tasks challenging.

Possible Causes and Triggers

The exact cause of fibromyalgia remains unknown, but research suggests it involves a combination of genetic, environmental, and psychological factors. It is believed that fibromyalgia amplifies painful sensations by affecting the way the brain processes pain signals. Triggers for fibromyalgia can include physical trauma, surgery, infection, or significant psychological stress. In some cases, symptoms gradually accumulate over time without a single triggering event.

The Diagnostic Process

Diagnosing fibromyalgia can be challenging because its symptoms overlap with other conditions. There is no specific lab test for fibromyalgia; instead, diagnosis is typically made based on a history of widespread pain lasting more than three months, combined with the presence of other symptoms such as fatigue and cognitive issues. Healthcare providers may use specific criteria, such as the 18 tender points, to aid in diagnosis, though newer guidelines emphasize the overall symptom severity and duration.

Impact on Daily Life
Living with fibromyalgia means adapting to a new normal. The unpredictability of symptoms can make planning daily activities difficult, and the chronic pain and fatigue can lead to frustration and emotional distress. However, understanding the condition and adopting effective management strategies can help improve the quality of life. This includes lifestyle changes, such as incorporating regular, gentle exercise, practicing stress management techniques, and maintaining a healthy diet.

Hope and Resilience
Despite its challenges, many people with fibromyalgia lead fulfilling lives. The key lies in finding the right combination of treatments and strategies that work for you. With the purpose of giving you hope and a path to resilience, this book seeks to arm you with the information and skills necessary to manage fibromyalgia. By sharing my personal experiences and comprehensive research, I hope to empower you to take control of your health and well-being, and to find strength in knowing you are not alone in this journey.

Fibromyalgia may be a part of your life, but it does not define you. With the right support, information, and determination, you can manage your symptoms and live a life full of purpose and joy. This book is here to guide you every step of the way.

DISPELLING FIBROMYALGIA MISCONCEPTIONS

Living with fibromyalgia is like navigating through a dense fog while carrying a backpack full of rocks. Every step is a challenge, every day a battle against an invisible enemy. But for millions of people living with this condition worldwide, the pain and fatigue are just the beginning of their struggle.

Imagine waking up each morning feeling like you've been hit by a truck, only to face a world that doubts your pain exists. This is the daily reality for those with fibromyalgia. The misconceptions surrounding this condition aren't just harmless misunderstandings; they're barriers that isolate, labels that wound, and obstacles that stand between sufferers and the help they desperately need.

As a society, we often pride ourselves on our compassion and understanding. Yet, when it comes to fibromyalgia, we often fall short. It's time to change that narrative. In this journey, we'll explore the most deeply rooted misconceptions about fibromyalgia. This isn't just about debunking myths; it's about building bridges of understanding and compassion in our communities, our healthcare systems, and our societies at large.

Because behind every misconception is a person fighting a battle most of us can't see – a person who deserves to be seen, heard, and understood for what they're truly experiencing. As we dive into these misconceptions, remember: this could be your neighbor, your coworker, your friend, or even a family member. Their struggle is real, and it's time we acknowledged it.

Misconceptions:

"It's Just Attention-Seeking Behavior" Think about the last time you had to cancel plans because you were sick. Now imagine doing that regularly, watching as your social circle slowly shrinks. For those with fibromyalgia, this is often their reality. They're not seeking attention; they're often forced to retreat from the spotlight. That empty chair at the family gathering or the absence at the office party isn't a cry for attention – it's a silent struggle against a body that won't cooperate. The next time you notice someone consistently missing from social events, consider that they might be fighting a battle you can't see.

"They're Just Lazy" In a world that often values productivity above all else, being labeled as 'lazy' is particularly hurtful. For someone with fibromyalgia, simply getting out of bed can feel like running a marathon. What looks like laziness to an outsider is often an immense, invisible effort. That colleague who always seems tired? They might have spent their entire energy reserve just making it to the office. It's time we redefined what strength looks like – sometimes, it's the person who shows up despite overwhelming odds.

"It's Just Stress" Sure, stress can make fibromyalgia symptoms worse, but saying it's the root cause is like saying a match caused a forest fire while ignoring the drought conditions. In our fast-paced modern life, stress is almost a given. But fibromyalgia goes beyond that. It's a complex interplay of neurological and physiological factors that scientists are still working to fully understand. Reducing it to "just stress" undermines the very real, physical nature of the condition.

"It's Just Depression" As mental health awareness grows globally, it's easy to lump fibromyalgia in with conditions like depression. While they can co-exist, they're not the same. Depression is a serious condition that deserves its own recognition and treatment, but so does the physical pain of fibromyalgia. Imagine telling someone with a broken leg that they're just sad. Sounds absurd, right? That's how it feels to have your chronic pain dismissed as "just depression."

"It's a Connective Tissue Disease" Our understanding of the human body is constantly evolving, and fibromyalgia is at the forefront of this evolution. Unlike connective tissue diseases, fibromyalgia doesn't cause visible damage to joints or tissues. It's more like a glitch in the body's pain processing system. This distinction is crucial for proper treatment and understanding. It's the difference between trying to fix a software problem with hardware solutions.

"Fibromyalgia Is Imaginary" In an age of scientific advancement, it's shocking that some still believe fibromyalgia isn't real. It's recognized by major medical institutions across the world. Telling someone their pain is imaginary is not just incorrect, it's disrespectful to their lived experience and the scientific community's findings.

"It's Hypochondria" There's a big difference between being overly worried about your health and living with chronic pain and fatigue. Hypochondria is a mental health condition, while fibromyalgia is a neurological disorder with very real physical symptoms. Confusing the two is like mistaking a fire alarm for the fire itself – one is a reaction, the other is a real, ongoing issue.

"It's an Autoimmune Disease" As autoimmune diseases become increasingly recognized, it's easy to lump fibromyalgia in with them. But fibromyalgia doesn't cause inflammation or tissue damage like autoimmune diseases do. Instead, it's more like the body's pain volume knob is stuck on high. Understanding this difference is crucial for proper treatment and research direction.

"It's Just a Mental Health Issue" Mental health is finally getting the attention it deserves, but that doesn't mean we should categorize all invisible illnesses as mental health conditions. Fibromyalgia has a strong neurological component. It's like the brain's pain processing center is working overtime, even when there's no apparent reason. This doesn't make it any less real or any less physical than a broken bone.

"There's No Visible Proof" In our evidence-based society, we often want concrete, visible proof. But not all real things can be seen or measured with our current tools. The absence of a simple diagnostic test doesn't negate the existence of fibromyalgia. It's like denying the existence of gravity just because you can't see it – you might not see it, but you can certainly feel its effects.

"It Only Affects Middle-Aged Women" Fibromyalgia can affect anyone – men, children, the elderly, people of all races and backgrounds. While it's more commonly diagnosed in middle-aged women, limiting our understanding to one demographic potentially leaves many sufferers undiagnosed and unsupported.

Conclusion

Dismantling these myths isn't just an academic exercise; it's a step towards a more compassionate and inclusive world. Every time we challenge one of these misconceptions, we open a door to better understanding, more focused research, and improved support for those living with fibromyalgia.

Imagine a world where invisible pain is acknowledged, where silent struggles are honored, where every person with fibromyalgia feels seen, heard, and supported. This is the world we should strive for.

Fibromyalgia is real, complex, and deserves our full attention and respect. It's not just a medical condition; it's a human journey of resilience, courage, and hope. As a global community, we have the power to come together to support those in need. Let's extend that same spirit to those battling fibromyalgia.

Let's continue to educate, support, and listen. Because what we're doing here isn't just debunking myths – we're building bridges of empathy that can transform lives. We're upholding the values of compassion and understanding that are at the heart of our shared humanity.

Remember, behind every diagnosis is a person, a story, a universe of experiences. And each of us has the power to make a difference, one act of understanding at a time. Let's create the opportunity for everyone to be understood and supported, regardless of the invisibility of their struggle.

Together, we can create a future where fibromyalgia is met with knowledge instead of skepticism, with support instead of stigma. Because that's who we are as human beings – we face challenges head-on, we support our neighbors, and we never stop striving for a better, more understanding world for all.

PART 1: UNDERSTANDING FIBROMYALGIA

Comprehending fibromyalgia is essential for effectively managing this intricate and frequently misinterpreted ailment. Fibromyalgia is a debilitating condition that causes fatigue, pain, and other symptoms that affect daily functioning. This condition, which affects millions of people worldwide, is still very difficult to detect and treat. Understanding fibromyalgia requires first defining it precisely and identifying its main symptoms. This encompasses not only the widespread pain that characterizes the illness but also the weariness, insomnia, and cognitive impairments that are frequently referred to as "fibro fog". Since the severity and frequency of these symptoms can differ widely, every person's experience with fibromyalgia is different.

A critical aspect of understanding fibromyalgia is exploring its causes and triggers. While the exact cause remains unknown, research has identified several contributing factors, including genetic predisposition, central sensitization, and environmental influences. Stress, physical trauma, and infections are also known to trigger or exacerbate symptoms. Recognizing these factors can help individuals identify and manage their personal triggers, leading to better symptom control.

Diagnosing fibromyalgia presents its own set of challenges. There is no single test to confirm the condition, so healthcare providers must rely on a combination of patient history, symptom assessment, and the exclusion of other disorders. The process often involves various lab tests and imaging studies to rule out conditions with similar symptoms. Accurate diagnosis is crucial for developing an effective treatment plan tailored to the individual's needs.

Finally, fibromyalgia is often associated with other chronic conditions. Common comorbidities include Irritable Bowel Syndrome (IBS), depression, anxiety, Chronic Fatigue Syndrome (CFS), and migraines. These associated conditions can complicate the clinical picture and require a comprehensive approach to treatment. In Part I of this book, we will delve into these essential aspects of fibromyalgia. By gaining a deeper understanding of what fibromyalgia is, what causes it, how it is diagnosed, and what other conditions are commonly associated with it, readers will be better equipped to manage their symptoms and improve their quality of life.

CHAPTER 1: WHAT IS FIBROMYALGIA?

The first step in comprehending fibromyalgia is realizing how complicated it is and how much of an influence it has on the lives of those who have it. Widespread physical pain, persistent exhaustion, and a host of other incapacitating symptoms are indicative of this disorder, which frequently interferes with everyday tasks and lowers quality of life. Even though fibromyalgia is one of the most prevalent chronic pain conditions, it is still largely unknown, which causes misunderstandings regarding its causes and characteristics.

The journey to recognize fibromyalgia as a legitimate medical condition has been long and fraught with challenges. For centuries, individuals suffering from this perplexing condition were often dismissed or misdiagnosed, as the medical community struggled to understand the mechanisms behind their pain. Early descriptions of similar conditions date back to the 19th century, but it wasn't until the late 20th century that significant strides were made in defining and diagnosing fibromyalgia.

This chapter delves into the essential aspects of fibromyalgia, starting with a clear definition and an exploration of its key symptoms. By examining the hallmark signs of the condition, such as widespread pain and tender points, we can better appreciate the daily struggles faced by those with fibromyalgia. Understanding these symptoms is crucial for recognizing the condition and seeking appropriate treatment and support.

Next, we explore the history and evolution of the diagnosis of fibromyalgia. From the early concepts of "muscular rheumatism" and "fibrositis" to the modern understanding of central sensitization, the path to recognizing fibromyalgia has been marked by significant advancements and shifts in perspective. These historical milestones highlight the dedication of researchers and clinicians in unraveling the complexities of fibromyalgia and paving the way for more effective management strategies.

In this chapter, we aim to provide a comprehensive overview of what fibromyalgia is, offering insights into its defining characteristics and the journey toward its recognition. By shedding light on both the clinical and historical aspects of fibromyalgia, we hope to foster a deeper understanding and empathy for those affected by this challenging condition.

DEFINITION AND KEY SYMPTOMS

The symptoms of fibromyalgia, a complicated and sometimes misdiagnosed illness, include fatigue and generalized discomfort. All over the body, it causes persistent pain and soreness, affecting the muscles and soft tissues. Although the exact etiology of fibromyalgia is still unknown, it is generally acknowledged that a mix of psychological, environmental, and genetic variables play a role in its development.

Widespread musculoskeletal pain is the primary symptom of fibromyalgia. Most people who have experienced this discomfort describe it as a dull aching that has persisted for at least three months. The pain has to be experienced on both sides of the body, above and below the waist, in order to be considered fibromyalgia. Many individuals with fibromyalgia report that the pain feels like a persistent flu-like ache or a deep muscular soreness.

In addition to widespread pain, fibromyalgia sufferers often experience **tender points**—specific areas of the body that are exceptionally sensitive to pressure. These tender points are commonly located in the neck, shoulders, back, hips, and knees. Even a slight touch in these areas can result in significant discomfort. The presence of these tender points is a key factor in diagnosing fibromyalgia.

Fatigue is another pervasive symptom that profoundly affects those with fibromyalgia. Unlike normal tiredness, the fatigue associated with fibromyalgia is often described as an overwhelming sense of exhaustion that interferes with daily activities. This fatigue can be both physical and mental, leading to a feeling of being constantly drained of energy. Many patients wake up feeling unrefreshed, even after a full night's sleep, and struggle with staying awake and alert throughout the day.

Cognitive difficulties, commonly referred to as "fibro fog," are another troubling aspect of fibromyalgia. Individuals with fibro fog often report problems with memory, concentration, and mental clarity. This can manifest as difficulty focusing, slowed thinking, and forgetfulness. These cognitive challenges can significantly impact the quality of life and make it difficult to perform everyday tasks, especially those requiring sustained attention or mental effort.

Sleep disturbances are also prevalent among those with fibromyalgia. Many patients experience non-restorative sleep, where they wake up feeling just as tired as when they went to bed. Conditions such as restless legs syndrome and sleep apnea are also more common in fibromyalgia patients, further disrupting their sleep patterns and exacerbating fatigue and pain levels.

Fibromyalgia often coexists with other chronic conditions, which can complicate diagnosis and treatment. These comorbid conditions include **irritable bowel syndrome (IBS)**, **migraines**, **interstitial cystitis**, **temporomandibular joint disorders (TMJ)**, and various mood disorders such as **depression** and **anxiety**. The overlapping symptoms of these conditions can make it challenging to identify and treat fibromyalgia effectively.

Sensitivity to stimuli is another notable symptom. People with fibromyalgia often report being unusually sensitive to lights, sounds, smells, and temperature changes. This hypersensitivity can make everyday environments feel overwhelming and can exacerbate other symptoms, including pain and fatigue.

Stiffness is a common morning complaint among fibromyalgia patients. Many individuals find that their muscles and joints are particularly stiff upon waking, which can make getting out of bed and starting the day particularly challenging. This stiffness can also occur after periods of inactivity, such as sitting or standing in one position for too long.

Numbness and tingling sensations, known as paresthesia, can also occur. These sensations often affect the hands and feet and can range from mild tingling to more severe numbness. While these symptoms can be alarming, they do not typically indicate nerve damage in fibromyalgia patients.

Mood disturbances are prevalent and can significantly impact overall well-being. Depression and anxiety are common, often exacerbated by chronic pain and fatigue. These mood disorders can create a vicious cycle, where pain and sleep disturbances worsen mental health, and poor mental health further exacerbates physical symptoms.

Understanding these key symptoms is crucial for recognizing and managing fibromyalgia. By identifying and addressing each symptom, individuals can better navigate their condition and work towards improving their quality of life.

HISTORY AND EVOLUTION OF THE DIAGNOSIS

The history of fibromyalgia is a fascinating journey marked by evolving understanding and shifting perspectives. This condition, often misunderstood and frequently misdiagnosed, has roots that trace back centuries, though its recognition as a distinct medical entity is relatively recent.

In the early 19th century, physicians documented cases of chronic pain syndromes that bore a striking resemblance to what we now recognize as fibromyalgia. Terms like "muscular rheumatism" were commonly used to describe these conditions, though the medical community lacked a clear understanding of their underlying mechanisms. Patients suffering from these ailments often faced skepticism and dismissal, as the concept of chronic pain without apparent physical damage was difficult for doctors to grasp.

The term "fibrositis" emerged in the early 20th century, suggesting an inflammatory process involving the fibrous tissues of the body. This term reflected the prevailing belief that inflammation was at the heart of the condition. However, as medical science advanced, it became evident that inflammation was not a consistent feature of the disorder. This realization led to a gradual shift in terminology and understanding.

Researchers started looking into how the central nervous system might be involved in chronic pain syndromes around the middle of the 20th century.

 This period saw the introduction of terms like "psychogenic rheumatism," highlighting the suspected psychological origins of the symptoms. While this perspective acknowledged the complexity of chronic pain, it also contributed to the stigma surrounding fibromyalgia, as patients were often perceived as suffering from a purely psychological issue.

The modern era of fibromyalgia research began in earnest in the 1970s and 1980s. During this time, Dr. Hugh Smythe, a pioneering rheumatologist, conducted extensive studies on patients with chronic widespread pain and tender points. His work laid the foundation for the American College of Rheumatology (ACR) to develop diagnostic criteria in 1990. These criteria included the presence of widespread pain for at least three months and tenderness in at least 11 of 18 specified tender points.

The ACR criteria represented a significant milestone in the recognition of fibromyalgia as a legitimate medical condition. However, the diagnostic process remained challenging, as the subjective nature of pain and tenderness made it difficult to establish a definitive diagnosis. Despite these challenges, the criteria provided a framework for further research and clinical practice, fostering greater awareness and understanding of the condition.

In the years that followed, fibromyalgia research continued to evolve. Advances in neuroimaging and neurobiology offered new insights into the central sensitization mechanisms underlying the disorder. Studies revealed abnormal pain processing pathways in the brains of fibromyalgia patients, shedding light on why they experience heightened pain sensitivity. These discoveries underscored the legitimacy of fibromyalgia as a neurological condition rather than a purely psychological one.

The American College of Rheumatology (ACR) revised its criteria for diagnosing fibromyalgia in 2010 to take into account the expanding body of research on the illness. The updated criteria moved the emphasis from tender sites to a more thorough evaluation of broad pain and related symptoms, including exhaustion, insomnia, and cognitive impairments. By using a comprehensive approach, the diagnosis accuracy was improved and the complex nature of fibromyalgia was captured.

Even with these developments, there is still more to learn about fibromyalgia. To fully understand the intricate interactions between genetic, environmental, and psychological factors that contribute to the illness, more research is required. With increasing understanding comes the possibility of better treatments and a higher standard of living for fibromyalgia sufferers. The history of fibromyalgia is a testament to the perseverance of patients and researchers alike, striving to bring clarity and compassion to a once-misunderstood disorder.

Conclusion

Fibromyalgia, marked by its myriad symptoms and complex history, has challenged patients and the medical community for centuries. Exploring its definition and key symptoms reveals the pervasive and often debilitating nature of this condition. Recognizing the widespread pain, chronic fatigue, and cognitive difficulties is crucial for effective management.

The historical journey toward the recognition of fibromyalgia highlights the evolving nature of medical understanding. From early misconceptions to modern advancements in neuroimaging and diagnostic criteria, the path to defining fibromyalgia reflects a growing acknowledgment of its legitimacy as a medical condition. These milestones underscore the importance of continued research and advocacy in improving the lives of those affected by fibromyalgia.

As we conclude this chapter, it is clear that while significant progress has been made, there is still much to learn about fibromyalgia. Our understanding of its causes, mechanisms, and effective treatments continues to evolve, driven by ongoing research and the experiences of those living with the condition. We can help create a more knowledgeable and helpful fibromyalgia management system by encouraging increased understanding and empathy, which will ultimately improve the lives of millions of people globally.

CHAPTER 2: CAUSES AND TRIGGERS

Unraveling the causes and triggers of fibromyalgia is a complex yet crucial endeavor in managing this challenging condition. For those living with fibromyalgia, understanding what exacerbates their symptoms can significantly impact their quality of life. While the exact cause of fibromyalgia remains a mystery, extensive research has highlighted several key theories and identified numerous triggers that can worsen symptoms. These insights offer a foundation for developing effective management strategies.

The scientific community has proposed various theories to explain the onset of fibromyalgia. Central sensitization is a leading theory, suggesting that the nervous system becomes hypersensitive, amplifying pain signals. This heightened sensitivity means that even minor stimuli can result in significant pain. Genetic predisposition is also believed to play a role, as fibromyalgia often runs in families, indicating that certain genetic markers might increase susceptibility to the condition. Additionally, neurotransmitter imbalances, particularly involving serotonin and norepinephrine, have been linked to fibromyalgia, affecting both pain perception and mood regulation.

Environmental and lifestyle factors are also significant. Physical or emotional trauma, stress, poor sleep quality, and infections are all potential contributors. These factors can interact with genetic and neurobiological predispositions to trigger or exacerbate fibromyalgia symptoms. Understanding the interplay between these various elements can help individuals identify their specific triggers and develop personalized strategies for managing their condition.

Identifying common triggers and learning how to manage them is a vital part of living with fibromyalgia. Stress, poor sleep, physical exertion, and dietary choices can all influence symptom severity. Environmental factors like weather changes and sensory inputs, as well as hormonal fluctuations and emotional stress, are also notable triggers. By recognizing these triggers, individuals can take proactive steps to mitigate their impact and improve their overall well-being.

This chapter delves into the current theories and scientific research surrounding the causes of fibromyalgia, followed by a detailed examination of common triggers and practical strategies for identifying and managing them. By gaining a deeper understanding of what influences fibromyalgia symptoms, individuals can better navigate their condition and work towards a more balanced and manageable lifestyle.

CURRENT THEORIES AND SCIENTIFIC RESEARCH

The quest to understand fibromyalgia has led to numerous theories and extensive scientific research, yet the exact cause remains elusive. What we do know is that fibromyalgia is a multifaceted condition, likely resulting from a combination of genetic, neurobiological, and environmental factors. This complex interplay creates a perfect storm, leading to the development and persistence of fibromyalgia symptoms.

Central Sensitization

One of the most prominent theories focuses on central sensitization. Central sensitization refers to a heightened sensitivity of the nervous system, making it overreact to stimuli that wouldn't normally cause pain. In individuals with fibromyalgia, the central nervous system, which includes the brain and spinal cord, amplifies pain signals. This means that even minor physical pressure or mild discomfort can be perceived as intense pain. Neuroimaging studies have shown that people with fibromyalgia have increased activity in pain-processing areas of the brain, supporting the central sensitization theory.

Genetic Predisposition

Genetic predisposition also plays a crucial role. Research has identified specific genetic markers that may increase the likelihood of developing fibromyalgia. These genetic variations can influence how pain is processed and how the body responds to stress. Family studies indicate that fibromyalgia tends to run in families, suggesting a hereditary component. People who have a family history of fibromyalgia or other chronic pain disorders may be more susceptible to getting the illness themselves.

Neurotransmitter Imbalances

Neurotransmitter imbalances are another area of interest. Neurotransmitters are chemicals in the brain that transmit signals between nerve cells. In fibromyalgia patients, levels of certain neurotransmitters, such as serotonin and norepinephrine, are often found to be abnormal. These neurotransmitters play a key role in mood regulation and pain perception. Imbalances can contribute to the heightened pain sensitivity and emotional disturbances commonly seen in fibromyalgia.

Stress and Trauma

The role of stress and trauma cannot be overlooked. Many individuals with fibromyalgia report a history of physical or emotional trauma, such as accidents, surgeries, or significant psychological stressors. These traumatic experiences have the potential to alter the body and brain, which can pave the way for the emergence of chronic pain disorders like fibromyalgia. Dysregulation of the hypothalamic-pituitary-adrenal (HPA) axis can result in chronic pain and exhaustion. The HPA axis regulates the body's reaction to stress.

Sleep Disturbances

Sleep disturbances are both a symptom and a potential cause of fibromyalgia. Poor sleep quality can exacerbate pain and fatigue, creating a vicious cycle where pain disrupts sleep, and lack of restorative sleep intensifies pain. Research indicates that deep sleep stages, crucial for physical and mental restoration, are often disrupted in fibromyalgia patients. This disruption can lead to an increase in pain sensitivity and other symptoms.

Inflammation

Inflammation has also been explored as a potential factor. While fibromyalgia is not considered an inflammatory disease, recent studies suggest that subtle inflammatory processes may be involved. Elevated levels of certain inflammatory markers have been found in some individuals with fibromyalgia. This low-grade inflammation might contribute to the symptoms and could explain why anti-inflammatory treatments offer relief to some patients.

Environmental Factors

Environmental factors such as infections or exposure to certain chemicals have been investigated for their potential role in triggering fibromyalgia. Infections caused by viruses like Epstein-Barr or Lyme disease bacteria have been linked to the onset of fibromyalgia in some cases. Similarly, exposure to environmental toxins or prolonged periods of physical inactivity may also contribute to the development of the condition.

Additional Potential Triggers

Although not fully established or confirmed by official medicine, several other potential triggers are believed to play a role in the development of fibromyalgia:

Environmental Pollution: Exposure to pollutants may exacerbate symptoms or trigger the onset of fibromyalgia.

Heavy Metal Poisoning: Toxic metals such as mercury, aluminum, and rhodium have been suggested as possible triggers.

Food Intolerances: Some individuals with fibromyalgia report that certain foods exacerbate their symptoms.

Intestinal Dysbiosis: An imbalance in the gut microbiome may contribute to systemic inflammation and pain.

Trauma: Both physical and emotional trauma can precipitate or worsen fibromyalgia symptoms.

Infections: Chronic infections, beyond those already mentioned, might play a role in triggering fibromyalgia.

Body's Toxic Load: The body's ability to detoxify, often linked to methylation problems, may influence the development of fibromyalgia. A high toxic load could exacerbate symptoms and overall health.

COMMON TRIGGERS AND HOW TO IDENTIFY THEM

Understanding the common triggers of fibromyalgia is essential for managing symptoms and improving quality of life. While the exact cause of fibromyalgia remains elusive, numerous triggers have been identified that can exacerbate symptoms. Recognizing and addressing these triggers can help individuals with fibromyalgia manage their condition more effectively.

Stress is a significant trigger for many people with fibromyalgia. Both physical and emotional stress can amplify the symptoms of fibromyalgia. Stress leads to the release of cortisol and other stress hormones, which can increase pain sensitivity and fatigue. Chronic stress can also disrupt sleep, which further exacerbates fibromyalgia symptoms. Learning stress management techniques such as mindfulness, meditation, and deep-breathing exercises can be beneficial.

Poor sleep quality is another common trigger. Many individuals with fibromyalgia suffer from sleep disturbances, including difficulty falling asleep, staying asleep, or achieving restorative sleep. Sleep deprivation can increase pain sensitivity and fatigue, creating a vicious cycle. Establishing a regular sleep routine, avoiding caffeine and electronics before bedtime, and creating a relaxing sleep environment can help improve sleep quality.

Physical exertion or inactivity can also trigger fibromyalgia symptoms. Overexertion can lead to muscle fatigue and pain, while prolonged inactivity can result in stiffness and increased pain sensitivity. Finding a balance between activity and rest is crucial. Gentle exercises such as yoga, tai chi, and swimming can help maintain mobility without overtaxing the muscles.

Weather changes and **temperature extremes** are known triggers for many with fibromyalgia. Cold, damp weather or sudden changes in weather can increase pain and stiffness. Extreme heat can also be problematic. Keeping warm during cold weather, using heating pads, and avoiding extreme temperatures can help manage these triggers.

Diet plays a role in triggering fibromyalgia symptoms. Certain foods and drinks can exacerbate symptoms, including those high in sugar, caffeine, and artificial additives. Alcohol and processed foods can also be problematic. Keeping a food diary can help identify which foods may be triggers. A balanced diet rich in whole foods, including fruits, vegetables, lean proteins, and whole grains, can support overall health and reduce symptom flare-ups.

Hormonal fluctuations can trigger fibromyalgia symptoms, particularly in women. Menstrual cycles, pregnancy, and menopause can all influence the severity of symptoms. Tracking hormonal changes and discussing them with a healthcare provider can help in managing these fluctuations.

Infections and illnesses can also act as triggers. Viral or bacterial infections can exacerbate symptoms, leading to increased pain and fatigue. Maintaining good hygiene, getting regular vaccinations, and seeking prompt treatment for infections can help minimize their impact.

Environmental factors such as loud noises, bright lights, and strong smells can trigger symptoms in some individuals with fibromyalgia. These sensory inputs can be overwhelming and increase pain sensitivity. Creating a calm, quiet environment and using tools such as noise-canceling headphones and sunglasses can help manage these triggers.

Emotional stress and psychological factors can significantly impact fibromyalgia symptoms. Anxiety, depression, and emotional trauma can all exacerbate symptoms. Seeking support through counseling, therapy, or support groups can provide emotional relief and help in managing these triggers.

Identifying and managing these common triggers can be challenging, but it is a crucial part of living with fibromyalgia. Keeping a detailed symptom diary can help track potential triggers and their impact on symptoms. By documenting daily activities, dietary intake, sleep patterns, and emotional states, individuals can begin to see patterns and identify specific triggers. Once identified, strategies can be implemented to minimize exposure to these triggers and manage their impact effectively.

Ultimately, managing fibromyalgia involves a multifaceted approach that includes recognizing and addressing these common triggers. By doing so, individuals can take proactive steps to reduce symptom flare-ups and improve their overall quality of life.

Conclusion

Understanding the causes and triggers of fibromyalgia is essential for effective management. Central sensitization, genetic predisposition, neurotransmitter imbalances, and environmental factors all contribute to the complexity of this condition. Recognizing the interplay between these elements provides a clearer picture of why symptoms occur and how they can be managed.

Identifying common triggers such as stress, poor sleep, physical exertion, dietary choices, and environmental factors empowers individuals to take control of their condition. By keeping a detailed symptom diary and observing patterns, patients can pinpoint specific triggers and develop personalized strategies to mitigate their effects. This proactive approach can lead to fewer symptom flare-ups and a better quality of life.

Navigating fibromyalgia involves a multifaceted approach, integrating scientific understanding with practical, everyday strategies. As research continues to uncover more about this condition, those affected can find hope in the growing knowledge and improved management techniques. By staying informed and proactive, individuals with fibromyalgia can lead more balanced and fulfilling lives.

CHAPTER 3: DIAGNOSING FIBROMYALGIA

Fibromyalgia diagnosis is a complex and frequently difficult procedure. In contrast to numerous medical diseases that can be detected with a single test or imaging study, fibromyalgia necessitates an interdisciplinary approach. The nature of the illness itself, which is marked by exhaustion, generalized pain, and a plethora of other symptoms that overlap with different conditions, is what causes this complexity. For those experiencing these symptoms, getting a proper diagnosis is crucial for effective management and treatment.

A comprehensive diagnostic process typically begins with a detailed medical history and symptom assessment. This involves understanding the patient's experience with pain, fatigue, sleep disturbances, and cognitive issues. A key part of this assessment is the identification of tender points, areas of the body that are particularly sensitive to pressure. Historically, the presence of tenderness in at least 11 out of 18 designated points was used to diagnose fibromyalgia. However, newer diagnostic criteria focus more on the overall pattern of widespread pain and the severity of accompanying symptoms.

Lab tests and other examinations play a critical role in ruling out other conditions that mimic fibromyalgia. Blood tests can help exclude conditions like rheumatoid arthritis, lupus, and thyroid disorders, all of which can present with similar symptoms. Imaging studies, such as X-rays, MRIs, and CT scans, are used to identify structural problems that could be causing pain. Additionally, sleep studies and psychological evaluations can provide valuable insights into other factors contributing to the patient's symptoms.

Being followed by a knowledgeable rheumatologist can make a significant difference in the diagnostic process. Rheumatologists specialize in musculoskeletal diseases and systemic autoimmune conditions, and their expertise can guide the selection of appropriate tests and evaluations tailored to the individual. This personalized approach ensures that all potential causes are thoroughly investigated, leading to a more accurate diagnosis and effective treatment plan.

By understanding the diagnostic process and the role of various tests and evaluations, patients and healthcare providers can work together to identify fibromyalgia and develop strategies to manage it effectively. This chapter will explore these elements in detail, providing a clear roadmap for navigating the complexities of diagnosing fibromyalgia.

DIAGNOSTIC PROCESS

Diagnosing fibromyalgia involves a comprehensive approach that considers the condition's unique characteristics. Unlike many medical conditions, it cannot be pinpointed through a single test or examination. Rather, it necessitates a thorough comprehension of the patient's medical background, symptom profile, and rule out any other possible reasons.

The first step in the diagnostic process typically involves a detailed **medical history**. A healthcare provider will inquire about the patient's symptoms, their duration, and how they impact daily life. They will also ask about any previous medical conditions, family history of chronic pain, and any recent physical or emotional trauma. This information helps to build a comprehensive picture of the patient's health and identifies patterns that might suggest fibromyalgia.

Symptom assessment is a critical component of diagnosing fibromyalgia. The primary symptom is **widespread pain**, which is usually described as a persistent, dull ache that lasts for at least three months. The discomfort needs to be felt above and below the waist, as well as on both sides of the body. The medical professional will also be on the lookout for additional symptoms that are frequently linked to fibromyalgia, like fatigue, sleep disruptions, and cognitive difficulties—sometimes known as "fibro fog."

A significant part of the diagnostic process is the identification of **tender points**. These are specific areas on the body that are extremely sensitive to pressure. Traditionally, the diagnosis of fibromyalgia required the presence of tenderness in at least 11 of 18 designated tender points. However, the diagnostic criteria have evolved, and the emphasis has shifted towards a more holistic evaluation of widespread pain and associated symptoms.

Exclusion of other conditions is crucial in the diagnostic process. Many other disorders can mimic the symptoms of fibromyalgia, including rheumatoid arthritis, lupus, and hypothyroidism. To rule out these and other conditions, healthcare providers often conduct various tests, including blood tests and imaging studies. These tests are not used to diagnose fibromyalgia directly but to eliminate other potential causes of the symptoms.

The American College of Rheumatology (ACR) has established specific **diagnostic criteria** to aid in the diagnosis of fibromyalgia. These criteria include a widespread pain index (WPI) and a symptom severity (SS) scale. The WPI assesses the extent and location of the pain, while the SS scale evaluates the severity of symptoms such as fatigue, waking unrefreshed, and cognitive issues. A combination of these scores helps to confirm the diagnosis of fibromyalgia.

Another important aspect of diagnosing fibromyalgia is the consideration of **coexisting conditions**. In addition to fibromyalgia, many people with this illness also have migraines, depression, and irritable bowel syndrome (IBS). Establishing a thorough treatment plan that takes into account every facet of the patient's health requires an understanding of these comorbidities.

The **patient's self-report** is an invaluable tool in the diagnostic process. Because fibromyalgia symptoms can be highly subjective, the patient's description of their pain and other symptoms provides critical insight. Healthcare providers may use questionnaires and pain diaries to gather detailed information about the patient's experience, which can aid in the diagnosis.

Diagnosing fibromyalgia is a nuanced and detailed process that requires careful consideration of multiple factors. The goal is not only to confirm the presence of fibromyalgia but also to understand the broader impact on the patient's life and to develop a tailored treatment plan. Through a combination of medical history, symptom assessment, exclusion of other conditions, and established diagnostic criteria, healthcare providers can accurately diagnose fibromyalgia and help patients manage this challenging condition.

LAB TESTS AND OTHER EXAMINATIONS

Fibromyalgia diagnosis is a complex process that includes a patient history, symptom assessment, and elimination of other illnesses. While there is no single test to definitively diagnose fibromyalgia, lab tests and other examinations play a crucial role in ruling out other potential causes of the symptoms. This process of exclusion helps ensure that a diagnosis of fibromyalgia is accurate and that other serious conditions are not overlooked.

Blood tests are often the first step in this diagnostic journey. These tests are not used to identify fibromyalgia directly but to eliminate other conditions that can mimic its symptoms. Common blood tests include a complete blood count (CBC), erythrocyte sedimentation rate (ESR), and C-reactive protein (CRP) test. These tests help detect inflammation and infection, which are not typical of fibromyalgia but are present in conditions like rheumatoid arthritis or lupus.

Another critical blood test is the **thyroid function test**. Hypothyroidism can cause symptoms similar to fibromyalgia, such as fatigue, muscle aches, and cognitive difficulties. By measuring levels of thyroid hormones (TSH, T3, and T4), doctors can determine if thyroid dysfunction is contributing to the patient's symptoms.

Vitamin D levels are also checked because vitamin D deficiency can lead to muscle pain and weakness. Low levels of this essential vitamin can exacerbate pain and fatigue, and supplementing vitamin D can alleviate these symptoms in some individuals.

In addition to blood tests, doctors may order **imaging studies** to further rule out other conditions. **X-rays**, **MRIs**, and **CT scans** can help detect structural abnormalities, such as arthritis, disc problems, or other musculoskeletal issues that could explain the patient's pain. While these imaging studies do not diagnose fibromyalgia, they are vital in ensuring that other potential causes of chronic pain are not missed.

Nerve conduction studies and **electromyography (EMG)** tests may be used if there are symptoms of numbness or tingling. These tests measure how well and how fast nerves can send electrical signals, helping to identify conditions like neuropathy or other neurological disorders that might be causing the symptoms.

Sleep studies can also be useful, particularly because sleep disturbances are common in fibromyalgia patients. Conditions such as sleep apnea or restless legs syndrome can be diagnosed through a polysomnogram, an overnight test that monitors brain activity, eye movements, heart rate, and muscle activity during sleep. Identifying and treating sleep disorders can significantly improve the overall well-being of a fibromyalgia patient.

Psychological evaluations may also be conducted, given the high prevalence of depression and anxiety in fibromyalgia patients. These evaluations help to understand the mental health aspects of the condition, which can inform a more comprehensive treatment plan. Tools such as the Beck Depression Inventory or the Hamilton Anxiety Rating Scale may be used to assess the severity of these conditions.

In some cases, doctors might use **specialized questionnaires** to gather detailed information about the patient's symptoms and their impact on daily life. The Fibromyalgia Impact Questionnaire (FIQ) and the Revised Fibromyalgia Impact Questionnaire (FIQR) are tools specifically designed to measure the health status and quality of life in people with fibromyalgia. These questionnaires address a wide range of symptoms, including pain, exhaustion, sleep difficulties, and psychological distress. The process of diagnosing fibromyalgia is thorough and multifaceted, involving various lab tests and examinations to rule out other conditions and confirm the diagnosis. While these tests cannot diagnose fibromyalgia on their own, they are essential in building a comprehensive understanding of the patient's health. By combining these diagnostic tools with clinical assessment and patient history, healthcare providers can arrive at a more accurate and confident diagnosis, paving the way for effective management and treatment.

Conclusion

Diagnosing fibromyalgia is a comprehensive and intricate process that requires a blend of clinical expertise, patient history, and diagnostic tests. While there is no single test to confirm fibromyalgia, a combination of symptom assessment, lab tests, and imaging studies helps rule out other conditions and supports a more accurate diagnosis. The involvement of a skilled rheumatologist can significantly enhance this process, ensuring that each patient receives a tailored evaluation that addresses their unique symptoms and medical history.

Understanding the various components of the diagnostic process empowers patients to actively participate in their healthcare journey. By being informed and proactive, individuals can collaborate effectively with their healthcare providers, leading to a clearer diagnosis and more effective management strategies. As research continues to evolve, the hope is that diagnosing fibromyalgia will become more straightforward, ultimately improving outcomes for those living with this challenging condition.

CHAPTER 4: CONDITIONS ASSOCIATED WITH FIBROMYALGIA

Living with fibromyalgia often means dealing with more than just widespread pain and fatigue. Many individuals with fibromyalgia also experience a range of other chronic conditions that complicate their symptoms and make management more challenging. These associated conditions can intensify the symptoms of fibromyalgia, creating a complex web of health issues that significantly impact daily life.

One of the most common comorbid conditions is **Irritable Bowel Syndrome (IBS)**, which causes abdominal pain, bloating, and changes in bowel habits. The connection between IBS and fibromyalgia is well-established, and many patients find that managing one condition helps alleviate the symptoms of the other. Similarly, **depression, anxiety** and **Short-term memory problems** are frequently seen in fibromyalgia patients. These disorders can exacerbate pain, fatigue, and other fibromyalgia symptoms, making it essential to address both the physical and psychological aspects of the condition.

Other conditions commonly associated with fibromyalgia include Chronic Fatigue Syndrome (CFS), migraines, Temporomandibular Joint Disorder (TMJ), Interstitial Cystitis (IC), and Restless Legs Syndrome (RLS). Each of these conditions brings its own set of challenges and can significantly impact a patient's quality of life. For example, the profound fatigue of CFS can compound the exhaustion already felt by fibromyalgia patients, while migraines and TMJ add additional layers of pain and discomfort.

Recognizing and understanding these associated conditions is crucial for developing an effective treatment plan. By identifying the full spectrum of symptoms and comorbidities, healthcare providers can tailor their approach to address all aspects of a patient's health. This comprehensive strategy not only helps manage fibromyalgia more effectively but also improves overall well-being.

This chapter delves into the conditions commonly associated with fibromyalgia, exploring their symptoms, impacts, and management strategies. By gaining a deeper understanding of these comorbid conditions, patients and healthcare providers can work together to develop more effective, holistic treatment plans that enhance the quality of life for those living with fibromyalgia.

IRRITABLE BOWEL SYNDROME (IBS)

Irritable Bowel Syndrome (IBS) is a common condition that frequently coexists with fibromyalgia. This chronic gastrointestinal disorder is characterized by a group of symptoms that include abdominal pain, bloating, and altered bowel habits such as constipation, diarrhea, or a mix of both. The connection between IBS and fibromyalgia is well-documented, and many individuals diagnosed with fibromyalgia also experience IBS, complicating their health picture and management strategies.

The relationship between fibromyalgia and IBS is multifaceted. Both conditions are believed to involve dysregulation of the central nervous system, leading to an increased sensitivity to pain. In fibromyalgia, this heightened sensitivity affects muscles and soft tissues, while in IBS, it impacts the gastrointestinal tract. This shared mechanism suggests that both conditions may be part of a broader syndrome of central sensitization, where the nervous system amplifies pain signals.

Symptoms of IBS can vary widely among individuals but often include chronic abdominal discomfort or pain, which is typically relieved by a bowel movement. Bloating and gas are also common, contributing to a feeling of abdominal distension. The altered bowel habits can be particularly distressing, as they are often unpredictable and can fluctuate between constipation and diarrhea. This variability can severely impact the quality of life, as individuals must constantly adapt to the changing nature of their symptoms.

The **impact of IBS on daily life** can be profound. Many people with IBS report that their symptoms interfere with their ability to work, socialize, and engage in regular activities. The unpredictability of the condition can lead to anxiety and stress, which in turn can exacerbate IBS symptoms, creating a vicious cycle. For those with fibromyalgia, managing both conditions simultaneously can be particularly challenging, as the symptoms of one can often trigger or worsen the symptoms of the other.

Managing IBS typically involves a combination of dietary changes, medications, and stress management techniques. Dietary modifications are often the first line of defense. Many individuals find relief by following a low-FODMAP diet, which involves reducing the intake of certain carbohydrates that are difficult to digest. Identifying and avoiding specific food triggers through an elimination diet can also be beneficial.

Medications can also play a role in managing IBS. Depending on the predominant symptoms, doctors may prescribe fiber supplements, laxatives, antidiarrheal medications, or antispasmodics. In some cases, low-dose antidepressants may be recommended to help modulate pain and improve bowel function.

Stress management is another crucial component in managing IBS. Mindfulness, meditation, and yoga are some techniques that can help reduce stress and its effects on the gastrointestinal system. Cognitive-behavioral therapy (CBT) has also been demonstrated to be useful in assisting individuals with managing the psychological aspects of IBS, such as anxiety and depression, which can aggravate physical symptoms.

For individuals with both fibromyalgia and IBS, a **multidisciplinary approach** is often necessary. Collaborating with healthcare providers who specialize in both conditions can help develop a comprehensive management plan. This might include working with a rheumatologist for fibromyalgia and a gastroenterologist for IBS, as well as incorporating support from nutritionists and mental health professionals.

Understanding the interplay between fibromyalgia and IBS is essential for effective management. By recognizing the connections between these conditions and addressing them holistically, individuals can achieve better control over their symptoms and improve their overall quality of life. With tailored strategies and comprehensive care, it is possible to navigate the complexities of living with both fibromyalgia and IBS.

DEPRESSION AND ANXIETY

Depression and anxiety are prevalent among individuals with fibromyalgia, profoundly affecting their overall well-being and complicating their management of the condition. The connection between fibromyalgia and these mental health disorders is well-documented, with research indicating that as many as 50% of those with fibromyalgia also experience significant depression or anxiety. Understanding this relationship is crucial for developing a holistic treatment plan that addresses both the physical and emotional aspects of fibromyalgia.

Depression in fibromyalgia patients is often characterized by persistent feelings of sadness, hopelessness, and a lack of interest or pleasure in activities once enjoyed. This can be compounded by the chronic pain and fatigue associated with fibromyalgia, which can limit physical activity and social interactions, further contributing to depressive symptoms. The physical limitations imposed by fibromyalgia can lead to a sense of loss and frustration, exacerbating feelings of depression.

Anxiety, on the other hand, manifests as excessive worry, nervousness, and fear. For those with fibromyalgia, anxiety can stem from the unpredictability of pain flare-ups and the impact this has on their daily lives. The constant anticipation of pain can create a heightened state of alertness, leading to chronic stress and anxiety. This can interfere with sleep, exacerbate pain, and create a cycle where anxiety and pain reinforce each other.

The relationship between fibromyalgia, depression, and anxiety is bidirectional. Chronic pain and fatigue can trigger depressive and anxious feelings, while these mental health conditions can intensify the perception of pain and the overall symptom burden. Neurobiological factors, such as imbalances in neurotransmitters like serotonin and norepinephrine, play a role in both fibromyalgia and mood disorders, suggesting a shared pathophysiology.

Managing depression and anxiety in fibromyalgia requires a comprehensive approach. **Psychotherapy**, particularly cognitive-behavioral therapy (CBT), has been shown to be effective in helping patients manage their symptoms. CBT focuses on changing negative thought patterns and behaviors, providing individuals with coping strategies to handle pain and improve their mood. Mindfulness-based stress reduction (MBSR) is another therapeutic approach that has proven beneficial, helping patients reduce stress and improve emotional regulation through mindfulness practices.

Medications can also be an important part of treatment. Antidepressants, including selective serotonin reuptake inhibitors (SSRIs) and serotonin-norepinephrine reuptake inhibitors (SNRIs), can aid with pain and mood issues. These medications work by balancing neurotransmitters in the brain, addressing both the physical and emotional aspects of fibromyalgia. Anti-anxiety medications might also be prescribed to manage severe anxiety symptoms.

Lifestyle modifications play an important part in managing depression and anxiety associated with fibromyalgia. Regular physical activity, tailored to the individual's abilities, can improve mood and reduce pain. Low-impact exercises such as walking, swimming, and yoga are particularly beneficial. A healthy diet, rich in nutrients, can support overall well-being and energy levels. Adequate sleep is also essential, as poor sleep can worsen both pain and mood issues. Techniques such as establishing a regular sleep routine and creating a relaxing bedtime environment can help improve sleep quality.

Support systems are vital for individuals with fibromyalgia. Connecting with others who understand the challenges of living with chronic pain can provide emotional support and practical advice. Support groups, either in-person or online, offer a community of individuals who can share their experiences and coping strategies.

For many patients, the combination of professional treatment, lifestyle changes, and a strong support network provides the best outcomes. The quality of life for people with fibromyalgia can be greatly improved by acknowledging and treating sadness and anxiety as essential parts of managing the difficult condition. By taking a holistic approach that addresses both the mind and body, individuals can achieve better control over their symptoms and improve their overall health.

SHORT-TERM MEMORY PROBLEMS

Short-term memory problems, often referred to as "fibro fog," are a common and particularly troubling symptom of fibromyalgia. These cognitive difficulties encompass a range of issues, including **problems with memory, concentration, and confusion**. Patients frequently report forgetting appointments, misplacing items, or struggling to find the right words during conversations. This cognitive impairment can significantly impact daily life, making it challenging to perform routine tasks, manage responsibilities, and maintain productivity.

"Fibro fog" is not merely an inconvenience; it can lead to serious disruptions in a person's personal and professional life. For instance, a patient might find it difficult to keep track of their work tasks, leading to decreased job performance. In social settings, memory lapses and confusion can cause embarrassment and strain relationships, as others might misinterpret these symptoms as a lack of attention or interest.

The exact cause of fibro fog is not fully understood, but it is believed to be linked to the overall dysfunction in the central nervous system associated with fibromyalgia. **Poor sleep quality**, which is common in fibromyalgia patients due to pain and other sleep disturbances, can exacerbate cognitive issues. Additionally, **chronic pain and fatigue** drain mental resources, making it harder to focus and remember details.

Managing fibro fog often requires a multifaceted approach. Ensuring good **sleep hygiene** is crucial; this can involve establishing a regular sleep schedule, creating a restful sleep environment, and addressing sleep disorders like sleep apnea or restless legs syndrome. **Cognitive exercises**, such as puzzles or memory games, can help keep the mind sharp. **Regular physical activity**, though challenging due to pain and stiffness, has been shown to improve both physical and mental health. **Stress management techniques**, including mindfulness, meditation, and therapy, can also alleviate some cognitive symptoms by reducing overall stress levels.

Medications used to treat fibromyalgia, such as certain antidepressants and anticonvulsants, may also help improve cognitive function indirectly by alleviating pain and improving sleep. It's essential for patients to work closely with their healthcare providers to develop a comprehensive treatment plan tailored to their specific needs. By addressing both the physical and cognitive aspects of fibromyalgia, patients can achieve better overall management of their symptoms and an improved quality of life.

INSOMNIA IN FIBROMYALGIA PATIENTS

Insomnia is a prevalent and distressing symptom among fibromyalgia patients, significantly impacting their overall well-being and quality of life. Characterized by difficulty falling asleep, staying asleep, or experiencing restorative sleep, insomnia can exacerbate the other symptoms of fibromyalgia, creating a vicious cycle of pain and fatigue.

Impact on Daily Life: The persistent lack of quality sleep can lead to severe fatigue, reduced cognitive function, and increased sensitivity to pain. This, in turn, affects patients' ability to perform daily tasks, maintain employment, and engage in social activities, contributing to a diminished quality of life.

Pain and Sleep Disruption: The chronic pain associated with fibromyalgia often prevents patients from finding a comfortable sleeping position, leading to frequent awakenings and difficulty staying asleep. This pain-induced sleep disruption exacerbates the overall discomfort and fatigue experienced by fibromyalgia patients.

Cognitive Impairment: Known as "fibro fog," cognitive impairments, including difficulty with memory, concentration, and decision-making, are often exacerbated by poor sleep quality. Insomnia intensifies these cognitive difficulties, making it even more challenging for patients to function effectively in their daily lives.

Emotional and Psychological Effects: Chronic insomnia can lead to or worsen mental health issues such as depression and anxiety, which are common comorbidities in fibromyalgia patients. The stress and frustration of not being able to sleep can heighten feelings of hopelessness and despair, further affecting mental health.

Immune System Dysfunction: Sleep is crucial for the body's immune function. Chronic insomnia can weaken the immune system, making fibromyalgia patients more susceptible to infections and illnesses, and can exacerbate the severity and frequency of fibromyalgia flares.

Hormonal Imbalances: Sleep disturbances can lead to hormonal imbalances, including disruptions in the production of cortisol and melatonin, which regulate stress and sleep-wake cycles. These imbalances can increase pain sensitivity and stress levels, contributing to the overall symptom burden in fibromyalgia patients.

Non-Restorative Sleep: Even when fibromyalgia patients manage to sleep, it is often non-restorative, meaning they do not wake up feeling refreshed. This lack of restorative sleep is a hallmark of fibromyalgia and significantly impacts patients' energy levels and ability to function during the day.

Management Strategies: Addressing insomnia in fibromyalgia patients requires a multifaceted approach. Cognitive-behavioral therapy for insomnia (CBT-I) has been shown to be effective in improving sleep quality. Medications such as low-dose antidepressants, gabapentinoids, or sleep aids may also be prescribed to help manage pain and improve sleep. Additionally, lifestyle modifications, such as establishing a regular sleep schedule, creating a restful sleep environment, and avoiding caffeine and electronics before bedtime, can also support better sleep hygiene.

Insomnia is a debilitating symptom of fibromyalgia that significantly impacts patients' physical, cognitive, and emotional health. Comprehensive management that addresses both sleep disturbances and the broader spectrum of fibromyalgia symptoms is essential to improve quality of life. By focusing on both pharmacological and non-pharmacological interventions, healthcare providers can help fibromyalgia patients achieve better sleep and, consequently, better overall health and well-being.

OTHER COMMON CONDITIONS

Fibromyalgia frequently coexists with other chronic conditions, complicating the lives of those affected. These comorbidities can intensify fibromyalgia symptoms, making management more challenging. Recognizing these associated conditions is crucial for comprehensive care.

Chronic fatigue syndrome (CFS), also known as myalgic encephalomyelitis (ME), is one such condition frequently seen alongside fibromyalgia. Like fibromyalgia, CFS is characterized by profound, unexplained fatigue that doesn't improve with rest and is often worsened by physical or mental activity. The overlap in symptoms, including joint pain, sleep disturbances, and cognitive issues, can make it difficult to distinguish between the two conditions. Patients with both fibromyalgia and CFS often experience an intense and persistent exhaustion that significantly impacts their quality of life.

Migraines and tension headaches Migraines and tension headaches are another common comorbidity in fibromyalgia patients, adding another layer of pain and discomfort. Frequent headaches, which can range from mild tension headaches to severe migraines, are often reported. Tension headaches typically feel like a tight band around the head, while migraines are characterized by throbbing pain on one side of the head. Migraines are often accompanied by increased sensitivity to light and sound, nausea, and visual disturbances like seeing flashing lights or blind spots. The chronic nature of these headaches can compound the daily struggles faced by fibromyalgia patients, significantly interfering with their quality of life. Managing these headaches effectively often requires a combination of medications, lifestyle changes, and stress reduction techniques to minimize their frequency and severity.

Temporomandibular joint disorder (TMJ) is also commonly associated with fibromyalgia. TMJ causes pain and dysfunction in the jaw joint and muscles controlling jaw movement. Symptoms include jaw pain, clicking or popping sounds when opening the mouth, and difficulty chewing. The pain from TMJ can radiate to the neck and shoulders, which can be particularly troublesome for those already dealing with widespread musculoskeletal pain from fibromyalgia.

Facial pain, particularly in the muscles and jaw, is a persistent issue for many with fibromyalgia. This pain is often linked to temporomandibular joint disorder (TMJ), which causes dysfunction in the jaw joint and muscles controlling jaw movement. Patients typically describe this pain as a dull, aching sensation that can radiate to the neck and shoulders, exacerbating the widespread musculoskeletal pain characteristic of fibromyalgia. The discomfort can make chewing difficult, and the jaw may produce clicking or popping sounds. Effective management of facial pain often involves a combination of dental treatments, physical therapy, and stress management techniques to alleviate the symptoms and improve quality of life.

Interstitial cystitis (IC), a chronic bladder condition causing bladder pressure, bladder pain, and sometimes pelvic pain, is frequently seen in those with fibromyalgia. Symptoms of IC can vary but often include a persistent, urgent need to urinate and painful urination. The pain and suffering brought on by IC can have a substantial impact on day-to-day activities and quality of life, aggravating the symptoms of fibromyalgia.

Restless legs syndrome (RLS) is another condition that commonly co-occurs with fibromyalgia. RLS causes an uncontrollable urge to move the legs, often accompanied by uncomfortable sensations. These symptoms typically worsen in the evening or night, disrupting sleep and leading to increased fatigue. Given that sleep disturbances are already a significant issue for those with fibromyalgia, the presence of RLS can further exacerbate fatigue and impact overall well-being.

Persistent muscle stiffness: Persistent muscle stiffness is a hallmark of fibromyalgia, particularly noticeable in the morning or after periods of inactivity. This stiffness can make movement difficult and increase overall pain levels. Patients often describe feeling as if their muscles are tight and unable to relax, which can limit their range of motion and reduce physical activity. The stiffness typically affects the entire body but is often most severe in the neck, shoulders, and lower back. To manage muscle stiffness, a combination of gentle stretching exercises, warm baths, physical therapy, and medications may be recommended. Regular physical activity, though challenging, can help reduce stiffness and improve overall function.

Carpal Tunnel Syndrome: Symptoms of carpal tunnel syndrome, such as tingling, numbness, and pain in the hands and wrists, are common among those with fibromyalgia. These symptoms often worsen at night, disrupting sleep and daily activities. Patients might experience difficulty gripping objects or performing tasks that require fine motor skills. Effective management may include wrist splints, physical therapy, and sometimes surgical intervention.

Sciatica: Pain that radiates along the sciatic nerve, which runs down one or both legs from the lower back, can be a frequent complaint in fibromyalgia patients. This pain can range from a dull ache to sharp, burning sensations and can significantly impair mobility. Physical therapy, medications, and exercises to strengthen the lower back and improve flexibility can help manage sciatica symptoms.

Leg Cramps: Sudden, painful cramps in the legs are a common occurrence among fibromyalgia patients. These cramps can disrupt sleep and daily activities, contributing to overall discomfort. Stretching exercises, adequate hydration, and electrolyte balance can help reduce the frequency and severity of leg cramps.

Numbness or Tingling (Paresthesia): Many fibromyalgia patients experience abnormal sensations such as tingling, pricking, or numbness in their extremities, known as paresthesia. These sensations can be uncomfortable and interfere with daily activities. Managing paresthesia often involves addressing the underlying fibromyalgia symptoms through medication, physical therapy, and lifestyle modifications.

Tinnitus (Ringing in the Ears): Persistent ringing in the ears can be both distracting and distressing for fibromyalgia patients. Tinnitus can interfere with concentration, sleep, and overall quality of life. Treatment options may include sound therapy, cognitive behavioral therapy, and medications to alleviate the symptoms.

Allergies (Hypersensitivity to Medications, Foods, and Pollutants): Increased sensitivity to various substances, including medications, foods, and environmental pollutants, is common in fibromyalgia patients. These sensitivities can cause allergic-like reactions and exacerbate symptoms. Identifying and avoiding triggers, along with working with a healthcare provider to manage reactions, is crucial.

Sleep Apnea: Beyond insomnia, sleep apnea and other sleep disturbances are common in fibromyalgia patients, contributing to overall fatigue and poor quality of sleep. Sleep apnea involves repeated interruptions in breathing during sleep, leading to daytime sleepiness and fatigue. Continuous positive airway pressure (CPAP) therapy, lifestyle changes, and addressing underlying fibromyalgia symptoms can improve sleep quality.

Sleep disorders are a prevalent and distressing issue for fibromyalgia patients, significantly affecting their overall well-being. Beyond insomnia, other sleep disturbances such as Restless Legs Syndrome (RLS) and sleep apnea are common among those with fibromyalgia. RLS causes an uncontrollable urge to move the legs, often accompanied by uncomfortable sensations, which typically worsen in the evening or at night, disrupting sleep. Sleep apnea, characterized by repeated interruptions in breathing during sleep, further compounds the problem by leading to poor sleep quality and chronic fatigue.

These disorders create a vicious cycle: poor sleep exacerbates the fatigue and pain associated with fibromyalgia, which in turn makes it harder to achieve restful sleep. The resulting sleep deprivation can lead to increased sensitivity to pain, cognitive difficulties, and a decline in daily functioning.

Dry Mouth (Sicca Syndrome): Chronic dryness of the mouth, known as Sicca syndrome, can cause significant discomfort in fibromyalgia patients. This dryness can lead to difficulties in speaking, swallowing, and increased risk of dental problems. Using saliva substitutes, staying hydrated, and maintaining good oral hygiene can help manage dry mouth symptoms.

Bruxism (Teeth Grinding): Many fibromyalgia patients suffer from bruxism, which is the grinding or clenching of teeth, particularly at night. This can lead to jaw pain, headaches, and dental issues. Management may include wearing a night guard, stress reduction techniques, and dental treatments.

Walking Difficulties: Pain and stiffness associated with fibromyalgia can make walking and other physical activities challenging. Patients might experience difficulty with balance, coordination, and endurance. Physical therapy, assistive devices, and tailored exercise programs can help improve mobility and reduce discomfort.

Neck Pain: Chronic pain in the neck area is a frequent symptom in fibromyalgia patients. This pain can be debilitating and limit the range of motion. Management strategies may include physical therapy, massage, medications, and ergonomic adjustments to daily activities.

Blood Circulation Issues: Poor blood circulation can lead to feelings of numbness and cold in the extremities, which is common in fibromyalgia patients. Keeping warm, gentle exercises, and medications that improve circulation can help alleviate these symptoms.

Ear Canal Itching and Excessive Earwax Production: Itching in the ear canals and increased earwax production can be bothersome for fibromyalgia patients. Managing these symptoms may involve regular ear cleaning and using ear drops to reduce irritation and wax build-up.

Unilateral Night Cramps: Painful cramps occurring predominantly on one side of the body at night can disrupt sleep and cause significant discomfort. Stretching before bed, staying hydrated, and ensuring proper electrolyte balance can help reduce the frequency of these cramps.

Difficulty in Communication and Expression: Patients with fibromyalgia may struggle with verbal expression and communication, often due to cognitive difficulties or pain-related distractions. Cognitive therapy, speech therapy, and supportive communication strategies can help improve these skills.

Chills Even at High Temperatures: Sensitivity to cold temperatures, even in warm environments, can be uncomfortable for fibromyalgia patients. Dressing in layers, using heating devices, and managing overall fibromyalgia symptoms can help manage this sensitivity.

Difficulty Climbing or Descending Stairs: Pain and stiffness can make navigating stairs particularly difficult for fibromyalgia patients. Using handrails, taking one step at a time, and engaging in exercises to strengthen the lower body can help improve mobility and safety.

Dysphagia (Difficulty Swallowing): Swallowing difficulties can arise in fibromyalgia patients, complicating eating and drinking. Management strategies may include speech therapy, dietary modifications, and addressing underlying muscle dysfunction.

Dysphonia (Voice Changes): Changes in voice quality, such as hoarseness, can occur in fibromyalgia patients. Voice therapy, staying hydrated, and avoiding vocal strain can help manage these symptoms.

Dyspareunia (Pain During Intercourse): Pain during intercourse is a significant issue for many women with fibromyalgia. Addressing this pain often involves pelvic floor therapy, lubricants, and open communication with partners to ensure comfort and intimacy.

Distorted Sensations: Abnormal sensory experiences, such as feeling like the skin is burning or crawling, are common in fibromyalgia patients. These sensations can be distressing and interfere with daily activities. Management may include medications, sensory integration therapy, and stress reduction techniques.

Conclusion

Navigating fibromyalgia is already challenging, but the presence of additional chronic conditions can make it even more complex. Recognizing and addressing these comorbid conditions—such as IBS, depression, anxiety, CFS, migraines, TMJ, IC, and RLS—is essential for comprehensive care. Each of these conditions can exacerbate the symptoms of fibromyalgia, creating a cycle of pain and discomfort that can be difficult to break.

A holistic approach that considers all associated conditions can significantly improve symptom management and overall quality of life. Collaborating with a multidisciplinary team of healthcare providers, including rheumatologists, gastroenterologists, mental health professionals, and others, can provide a tailored treatment plan that addresses the unique needs of each patient.

By understanding the interconnected nature of fibromyalgia and its common comorbidities, patients can take proactive steps to manage their symptoms more effectively. This comprehensive approach not only alleviates physical discomfort but also supports mental and emotional well-being, leading to a more balanced and fulfilling life.

UNCOMMON SYMPTOMS

While fibromyalgia is often associated with widespread pain, fatigue, and other well-known symptoms, there are also a variety of less common symptoms that can significantly impact the lives of those affected. Recognizing these uncommon symptoms is crucial for comprehensive management and improved quality of life for fibromyalgia patients.

Raynaud's Phenomenon: This condition causes some areas of the body, such as fingers and toes, to feel numb and cold in response to cold temperatures or stress. Raynaud's Phenomenon occurs due to smaller arteries that supply blood to the skin constricting excessively, limiting blood supply to affected areas. For individuals with fibromyalgia, this can add another layer of discomfort and complication to their condition. Management includes keeping warm, stress reduction, and medications that improve blood flow.

Hair Loss: Unexplained hair loss can be an alarming symptom for those with fibromyalgia. This can occur due to the stress and hormonal imbalances associated with chronic pain and fatigue. While not everyone with fibromyalgia will experience hair loss, it is a notable symptom that can affect self-esteem and emotional well-being. Addressing underlying causes, stress management, and using gentle hair care practices can help mitigate hair loss.

Sensitivity to Sound (Hyperacusis): Individuals with fibromyalgia may find themselves unusually sensitive to everyday sounds. This condition, known as hyperacusis, can make normal auditory experiences uncomfortable or even painful. Managing this symptom often requires creating a quiet and calm environment to minimize discomfort. Management strategies can include sound therapy, ear protection, and creating a quiet living environment.

Non-Cardiac Chest Pain (Costochondritis): Costochondritis involves inflammation of the cartilage that connects a rib to the breastbone, causing sharp, aching pain in the chest. This pain can mimic that of a heart attack, leading to significant anxiety and stress for the patient. Understanding that this is a common symptom of fibromyalgia can help alleviate some of that concern. Pain management techniques, anti-inflammatory medications, and gentle stretching can help alleviate symptoms.

Dry Eyes: Chronic dryness of the eyes can cause significant discomfort, often managed with artificial tears and staying hydrated. Regular eye exams and avoiding eye strain are also important.

Sudden Food Sensitivities: New sensitivities or intolerances to certain foods can cause gastrointestinal distress in fibromyalgia patients. Identifying and avoiding trigger foods, working with a nutritionist, and managing overall digestive health are key strategies.

Vision Problems: Blurred vision, difficulty focusing, and eye pain can also be symptoms of fibromyalgia. These visual disturbances can interfere with daily tasks and overall quality of life. Regular eye check-ups, using corrective lenses, and managing underlying fibromyalgia symptoms can help improve vision issues.

Vestibular Complaints: Dizziness, balance issues, and vertigo are not uncommon in fibromyalgia patients. These symptoms can be disorienting and increase the risk of falls and injuries. Vestibular rehabilitation therapy, medications, and lifestyle modifications can help manage these symptoms.

Myofascial Pain: This type of pain occurs when pressure on sensitive points in the muscles causes pain in seemingly unrelated parts of the body. It can be particularly severe and difficult to manage. Treatment often includes physical therapy, trigger point injections, and relaxation techniques.

Skin Complaints: Various skin issues, including rashes, itching, and increased sensitivity to touch, can occur in fibromyalgia patients. Keeping the skin moisturized, avoiding irritants, and using medications to manage skin symptoms are important.

Weight Fluctuations: Unexplained weight gain or loss due to hormonal imbalances, changes in activity levels, or medication side effects is common in fibromyalgia patients. Regular monitoring of weight, balanced nutrition, and working with healthcare providers to manage medication side effects are essential.

Menstrual and Groin Pain: More severe menstrual cramps and pelvic pain in women with fibromyalgia can be challenging. Pain management strategies, hormonal treatments, and lifestyle modifications can help alleviate symptoms.

Respiratory Muscle Dysfunction: Difficulty breathing or a sensation of chest tightness can lead to increased anxiety in fibromyalgia patients. Breathing exercises, respiratory therapy, and managing anxiety can help improve respiratory function.

Night Sweats and Cold Sensitivity: Sudden night sweats and extreme sensitivity to cold temperatures are common in fibromyalgia patients. Dressing in layers, using climate control in the bedroom, and managing overall fibromyalgia symptoms can help alleviate these issues.

Nausea and Digestive Issues: Beyond IBS, symptoms like nausea, slow digestion, and constipation can significantly affect appetite and nutritional intake in fibromyalgia patients. Dietary adjustments, medications, and working with a gastroenterologist can help manage these symptoms.

Lightheadedness and Dizziness: Frequent episodes of lightheadedness or feeling faint can pose a risk of falls in fibromyalgia patients. Staying hydrated, managing blood pressure, and avoiding sudden movements can help reduce these symptoms.

Chemical Sensitivity: Increased sensitivity to odors, chemicals, and pollutants can cause allergic-like reactions in fibromyalgia patients. Identifying and avoiding triggers, using air purifiers, and working with healthcare providers to manage reactions are essential.

Conclusion

The spectrum of symptoms experienced by individuals with fibromyalgia is broad and varied, extending beyond the common symptoms of pain and fatigue. Recognizing and understanding these less common symptoms is essential for a holistic approach to treatment. Healthcare professionals can provide more comprehensive care that improves symptom management and quality of life for fibromyalgia patients by treating all facets of the condition.

For those living with fibromyalgia, awareness and acknowledgment of these uncommon symptoms can help in seeking appropriate treatment and support. Comprehensive management that considers all possible symptoms can significantly enhance the well-being of fibromyalgia patients.

By expanding the understanding of fibromyalgia to include these less common symptoms, both patients and healthcare providers can work together to develop more effective, individualized treatment plans. For those managing this difficult disease, a more comprehensive approach is essential to enhancing their overall quality of life.

CONCLUSION TO PART I: UNDERSTANDING FIBROMYALGIA

Understanding fibromyalgia involves more than just recognizing its symptoms. It requires a comprehensive approach that considers the condition's multifaceted nature. This includes exploring the various theories about its causes, identifying common triggers, and acknowledging the challenges of diagnosis. Each of these elements is crucial for developing effective management strategies.

The diagnostic process for fibromyalgia is intricate and requires careful consideration of multiple factors. Healthcare providers must evaluate a patient's medical history, perform thorough symptom assessments, and use lab tests to rule out other conditions. This detailed approach ensures that patients receive an accurate diagnosis, which is the foundation for effective treatment.

Fibromyalgia often coexists with other chronic conditions, adding layers of complexity to patient care. Conditions like IBS, depression, anxiety, and migraines can exacerbate fibromyalgia symptoms and complicate treatment plans. Acknowledging these comorbidities and integrating their management into a holistic treatment plan is essential for improving patient outcomes.

As we conclude Part I, it is clear that understanding fibromyalgia is an ongoing journey. Advances in research continue to shed light on this condition, offering hope for better diagnostic tools and more effective treatments. By staying informed and proactive, individuals with fibromyalgia can take charge of their health, work closely with their healthcare providers, and find strategies that work best for them. In the following sections, we will build on this foundational knowledge, exploring practical approaches to managing fibromyalgia and improving overall well-being. Through a combination of medical treatment, lifestyle adjustments, and support, those living with fibromyalgia can achieve a better quality of life.

PART 2: MEAL PLANS AND RECIPES

Welcome to Part II: Meal Plans and Recipes, a comprehensive guide designed to help you navigate the path to better health through thoughtful, nutritious eating. This section includes a detailed 5-week meal plan and a variety of delicious recipes specifically tailored to support individuals with fibromyalgia. By following these plans and recipes, you will be providing your body with the essential nutrients it needs to reduce inflammation and improve your overall well-being.

At first, the 5-week meal plan and the array of recipes might seem overwhelming. It's completely normal to feel this way. However, with time and practice, these new eating habits will become second nature. The key is to take it one step at a time and be patient with yourself. As you incorporate these changes into your daily routine, you'll find that healthy eating becomes an automatic, effortless part of your life.

Use the 5-week meal plan as a roadmap to guide your nutritional journey. Each week focuses on different aspects of health, from detoxing and cleansing to reducing inflammation and boosting energy. The recipes provided are not only nutritious but also flavorful and satisfying, ensuring you enjoy every meal. Embrace the process, knowing that each step brings you closer to a healthier, more vibrant you.

CHAPTER 5: NUTRITION AND FIBROMYALGIA

The management of fibromyalgia, a syndrome marked by fatigue, extensive pain, and other incapacitating symptoms, is heavily dependent on nutrition. While there is no one-size-fits-all diet for those with fibromyalgia, understanding the connection between food and symptoms can significantly improve quality of life. The foods we consume can influence inflammation, pain perception, energy levels, and overall well-being.

The foundation of a fibromyalgia-friendly diet begins with **basic nutritional principles**. These include eating a variety of whole foods, staying hydrated, and balancing meals to ensure sustained energy throughout the day. Whole foods include necessary nutrients that support body functioning and help reduce inflammation. Examples of these foods include fruits, vegetables, lean meats, whole grains, and healthy fats. Adequate hydration is crucial for maintaining energy levels and cognitive function, both of which are often compromised in fibromyalgia patients. Balanced meals that include carbohydrates, proteins, and fats help stabilize blood sugar levels, preventing energy dips and mood swings.

Knowing which **foods to avoid and include** is another critical aspect of managing fibromyalgia. Processed foods, sugary items, artificial sweeteners, and excessive caffeine can exacerbate symptoms by promoting inflammation and disrupting sleep patterns. On the other hand, including whole grains, lean meats, fresh produce, healthy fats, and low-fat dairy products can help lower inflammation, promote muscle healing, and enhance general health. Foods rich in antioxidants and anti-inflammatory properties are particularly beneficial.

Understanding the **scientific explanations** behind these dietary impacts can further empower individuals with fibromyalgia to make informed choices. Research indicates that inflammation, oxidative stress, gut health, blood sugar regulation, neurotransmitter function, and nutrient deficiencies all play roles in fibromyalgia symptoms. For instance, anti-inflammatory foods can help manage pain, while foods high in fiber and probiotics support gut health and reduce systemic inflammation. Additionally, maintaining stable blood sugar levels and ensuring adequate intake of key nutrients like magnesium can help alleviate fatigue and muscle pain.

This chapter delves into these critical areas, offering a comprehensive guide to how nutrition can be harnessed to manage fibromyalgia symptoms effectively. By understanding and applying these principles, individuals with fibromyalgia can take proactive steps to improve their health and enhance their quality of life.

BASIC NUTRITIONAL PRINCIPLES

Nutrition plays a vital role in managing fibromyalgia symptoms and enhancing overall well-being. For individuals with fibromyalgia, maintaining a balanced and nutrient-rich diet can help mitigate pain, reduce inflammation, and improve energy levels. While there is no one-size-fits-all diet for fibromyalgia, certain nutritional principles can guide patients toward making healthier food choices that support their condition.

A fundamental aspect of good nutrition is **eating a variety of whole foods**. Nutrients found in whole foods—fruits, vegetables, lean meats, whole grains, and healthy fats—support and enhance body processes and overall health. These foods can help lower inflammation and strengthen the immune system since they are high in vitamins, minerals, antioxidants, and fiber. Including a wide range of colorful fruits and vegetables in the diet ensures a broad spectrum of nutrients.

Hydration is another key principle. Staying well-hydrated is crucial for overall health and can help reduce fatigue and improve cognitive function, which are often impaired in fibromyalgia patients. Drinking adequate amounts of water throughout the day helps maintain bodily functions and can prevent dehydration, which can exacerbate symptoms.

Balanced meals are essential for stabilizing blood sugar levels and providing sustained energy. For fibromyalgia patients, this means incorporating a mix of carbohydrates, proteins, and fats into each meal. Carbohydrates should come from whole grains, fruits, and vegetables rather than refined sugars and processed foods. Proteins, from sources such as lean meats, fish, legumes, and nuts, are crucial for muscle repair and immune function. Healthy fats, like those found in avocados, olive oil, and fatty fish, support brain health and reduce inflammation.

Portion control is important to avoid overeating, which can lead to weight gain and increased pressure on the joints, exacerbating pain. Eating smaller, more frequent meals can help maintain energy levels and prevent the fatigue that often accompanies fibromyalgia. Mindful eating practices, such as paying attention to hunger and fullness cues and eating slowly, can help with portion control and improve digestion.

Limiting processed foods and additives is another critical aspect of nutrition for fibromyalgia. Processed foods often contain high levels of sugar, unhealthy fats, and artificial additives that can trigger inflammation and worsen symptoms. Instead, focusing on fresh, whole foods can help manage symptoms more effectively.

Incorporating these basic nutritional principles into daily life can make a significant difference for individuals with fibromyalgia. By prioritizing whole foods, hydration, balanced meals, portion control, and minimizing processed foods, patients can better manage their symptoms and improve their overall quality of life. This holistic approach to nutrition not only supports physical health but also contributes to mental and emotional well-being, creating a comprehensive strategy for managing fibromyalgia.

FOODS TO AVOID FOR FIBROMYALGIA MANAGEMENT

Living with fibromyalgia requires a thoughtful approach to diet, as certain foods can exacerbate symptoms such as pain, fatigue, and digestive issues. In this subchapter, we will explore the key categories of foods to avoid, providing detailed explanations and examples to help you make informed choices for better health and symptom management.

While there is no cure for fibromyalgia, dietary choices play a significant role in managing symptoms. Certain foods can trigger inflammation, disrupt sleep, and contribute to overall discomfort. By avoiding these foods, individuals with fibromyalgia can reduce flare-ups and improve their quality of life.

Processed Foods

Processed foods are often laden with unhealthy fats, refined sugars, and artificial additives, all of which can increase inflammation and worsen fibromyalgia symptoms. These foods typically offer little nutritional value and can lead to increased pain and fatigue.

Examples:

- Fast food (e.g., burgers, fries)
- Snacks (e.g., chips, pretzels)
- Microwave meals (e.g., frozen dinners)
- Packaged desserts (e.g., cookies, cakes)
- Instant noodles
- Deli meats
- Canned soups
- Frozen pizzas
- Pre-packaged sauces

SUGARY DRINKS

Sugary drinks cause rapid spikes and crashes in blood sugar levels, contributing to fatigue and mood swings. These beverages are high in calories but low in nutritional value, making them particularly problematic for fibromyalgia sufferers.

Examples:

- Sodas
- Energy drinks
- Sweetened iced teas
- Fruit punches
- Lemonade
- Sports drinks
- Sweetened coffee drinks
- Flavored milk
- Tonic water
- Sweetened coconut water

Red Meat and Processed Meats

Red meat and processed meats are high in saturated fats and can promote inflammation. Regular consumption of these meats can exacerbate pain and contribute to other health issues such as heart disease.
Examples:

- Beef
- Pork
- Lamb
- Bacon
- Sausages
- Hot dogs
- Ham
- Salami
- Corned beef
- Deli meats

Refined Grains

Refined grains lack the fiber and nutrients found in whole grains, leading to rapid increases in blood sugar levels. This can result in increased fatigue and a potential worsening of fibromyalgia symptoms.
Examples:

- White bread
- Pasta
- White rice
- Pastries
- Muffins
- Cakes
- Cookies
- Pancakes
- Waffles
- Crackers

Trans Fats

Trans fats are found in many processed and fried foods and are known to increase inflammation, potentially leading to heightened fibromyalgia symptoms. Avoiding these fats is crucial for managing pain and overall health.
Examples:

- Margarine
- Fried foods
- Baked goods with hydrogenated oils
- Snack foods
- Frozen dinners

- Non-dairy coffee creamers
- Microwave popcorn
- Shortening
- Store-bought pie crusts
- Fast food fries

Dairy Products

Dairy products can cause digestive issues and inflammation in some people with fibromyalgia. While not everyone is sensitive to dairy, it can be beneficial to monitor your symptoms and consider dairy alternatives if necessary.
Examples:

- Milk
- Cheese
- Yogurt
- Butter
- Cream
- Ice cream
- Cottage cheese
- Sour cream
- Cream cheese
- Powdered milk

Artificial Sweeteners and Additives

Artificial sweeteners and additives can trigger fibromyalgia symptoms such as pain and fatigue. Choosing natural sweeteners and avoiding products with artificial additives can help mitigate these effects.
Examples:

- Aspartame
- Sucralose
- Saccharin
- High fructose corn syrup
- MSG
- Artificial colors
- Artificial flavors
- Preservatives
- Emulsifiers
- Texturizers

Alcohol and Caffeinated Beverages

Alcohol and caffeine can disrupt sleep and exacerbate fatigue and pain in fibromyalgia patients. Moderation is key, as both can lead to a temporary energy boost followed by a significant crash.
Examples:

- Beer
- Wine
- Spirits
- Cocktails
- Coffee
- Black tea
- Soda with caffeine
- Energy drinks
- Pre-workout drinks
- Caffeinated water

Conclusion

Managing fibromyalgia through diet involves making mindful choices to avoid foods that can trigger inflammation, pain, and fatigue. By steering clear of processed foods, sugary drinks, red meat, refined grains, trans fats, dairy products, artificial sweeteners, and excessive alcohol and caffeine, individuals with fibromyalgia can improve their symptoms and enhance their overall well-being.

FOODS TO EAT FOR FIBROMYALGIA MANAGEMENT

Managing fibromyalgia effectively involves more than just medication and exercise; diet plays a crucial role. Certain foods can help reduce inflammation, improve energy levels, and support overall health, which is particularly important for individuals suffering from fibromyalgia. This subchapter will delve into the best foods to include in your diet, providing detailed explanations and examples for each category to help you make informed and beneficial dietary choices.

Fresh Vegetables

Fresh vegetables are a cornerstone of a fibromyalgia-friendly diet. They are rich in vitamins, minerals, antioxidants, and fiber, all of which help reduce inflammation and support the immune system.
Examples:

- **Leafy Greens:** Spinach, kale, arugula, Swiss chard, collard greens.
- **Cruciferous Vegetables:** Broccoli, cauliflower, Brussels sprouts, cabbage.
- **Root Vegetables:** Carrots, sweet potatoes, beets.
- **Others:** Bell peppers, zucchini, tomatoes, cucumbers.

Fruits

Fruits are another essential component, providing natural sugars, fiber, vitamins, and antioxidants. They help to reduce inflammation and support overall health.
Examples:

- **Berries:** Blueberries, strawberries, raspberries, blackberries.
- **Citrus:** Oranges, lemons, limes, grapefruits.

- **Other Fruits:** Apples, pears, bananas, mangoes, pineapples, grapes, kiwi, peaches.

Lean Proteins

Lean proteins are vital for muscle repair and energy maintenance. They provide the necessary building blocks for maintaining muscle mass and supporting overall health.
Examples:

- **Poultry:** Chicken, turkey.
- **Fish:** Salmon, mackerel, tuna, sardines.
- **Plant-Based:** Tofu, tempeh, lentils, beans, chickpeas.
- **Others:** Eggs, Greek yogurt.

Whole Grains

Whole grains offer sustained energy and are high in fiber, which aids digestion and helps stabilize blood sugar levels, preventing energy dips and mood swings.
Examples:

- **Popular Choices:** Quinoa, brown rice, oats, whole wheat.
- **Ancient Grains:** Barley, farro, bulgur, millet, spelt, buckwheat.

Healthy Fats

Healthy fats are crucial for reducing inflammation and supporting brain health. They should be a regular part of the diet to improve both physical and mental well-being.
Examples:

- **Oils:** Olive oil, coconut oil, flaxseed oil.
- **Nuts and Seeds:** Walnuts, chia seeds, hemp seeds, almonds.
- **Others:** Avocado, fatty fish (such as salmon and mackerel), dark chocolate.

Nuts and Seeds

Nuts and seeds are rich in healthy fats, protein, and fiber. They help reduce inflammation and support overall health.
Examples:

- **Nuts:** Almonds, walnuts, pecans, hazelnuts, pistachios, cashews.
- **Seeds:** Chia seeds, flaxseeds, pumpkin seeds, sunflower seeds.

Anti-Inflammatory Spices

Spices not only add flavor to your meals but also have anti-inflammatory properties that can help manage fibromyalgia symptoms.

Examples:

- **Turmeric**
- **Ginger**
- **Cinnamon**
- **Garlic**
- **Cayenne Pepper**
- **Black Pepper**
- **Cumin**
- **Coriander**
- **Rosemary**
- **Basil**

Herbal Teas and Water

Staying hydrated is essential, and herbal teas can provide additional anti-inflammatory benefits. They can also help soothe digestive issues and improve overall well-being.

Examples:

- **Herbal Teas:** Chamomile tea, peppermint tea, green tea, rooibos tea, ginger tea, hibiscus tea, dandelion tea, fennel tea, lemon balm tea, nettle tea.
- **Water:** Ensure you drink plenty of plain water throughout the day to stay hydrated and support bodily functions.

Detailed Examples and Benefits

1. **Leafy Greens:** Spinach and kale are high in magnesium, a mineral that can help relax muscles and reduce pain.

2. **Berries:** Blueberries and strawberries are rich in antioxidants, which help combat oxidative stress and inflammation.

3. **Salmon:** This fatty fish is loaded with omega-3 fatty acids, which have powerful anti-inflammatory effects.

4. **Quinoa:** A complete protein and a good source of fiber, quinoa helps stabilize blood sugar levels and provides sustained energy.

5. **Olive Oil:** Rich in monounsaturated fats and antioxidants, olive oil helps reduce inflammation and supports heart health.

6. **Chia Seeds:** These tiny seeds are packed with omega-3 fatty acids, fiber, and protein, making them a great addition to any diet.

7. **Turmeric:** Contains curcumin, a compound with strong anti-inflammatory and antioxidant properties.

8. **Green Tea:** Offers a wealth of antioxidants and has anti-inflammatory properties that can help reduce fibromyalgia symptoms.

9. **Peppermint Tea:** Known for its soothing effects on the digestive system, which can be beneficial for those with fibromyalgia-related digestive issues.

Conclusion

A diet rich in fresh vegetables, fruits, lean proteins, whole grains, healthy fats, nuts, seeds, anti-inflammatory spices, and herbal teas can significantly aid in managing fibromyalgia symptoms. By incorporating these foods into your daily meals, you can help reduce inflammation, improve energy levels, and support overall health, making it easier to manage this chronic condition. Tailoring your diet to include these beneficial foods is a powerful step towards holistic fibromyalgia management.

SCIENTIFIC EXPLANATION OF FOOD IMPACT ON SYMPTOMS

The relationship between diet and fibromyalgia symptoms is complex and multifaceted. Scientific research has increasingly shown that what we eat can significantly influence our body's inflammatory responses, pain perception, and overall health. Understanding the scientific basis of how certain foods impact fibromyalgia symptoms can empower patients to make informed dietary choices.

Inflammation is a key factor in fibromyalgia. While fibromyalgia is not an inflammatory disease in the traditional sense, inflammation can exacerbate its symptoms. Certain foods are known to promote inflammation in the body, leading to increased pain and fatigue. For instance, diets high in sugar, refined carbohydrates, and trans fats can elevate inflammatory markers, worsening fibromyalgia symptoms. On the other hand, anti-inflammatory foods including fatty fish, fruits, vegetables, nuts, and seeds can aid in symptom relief and inflammation reduction.

Oxidative stress also plays a role in fibromyalgia. This occurs when there is an imbalance between free radicals and antioxidants in the body, leading to cell damage. Foods rich in antioxidants, such as berries, leafy greens, and nuts, can combat oxidative stress by neutralizing free radicals. Incorporating these foods into the diet can help protect the body's cells and reduce symptom severity.

Gut health is another crucial aspect. The gut microbiome, which consists of trillions of microorganisms, has a profound impact on overall health, including the immune system and inflammation. A healthy gut microbiome can help manage fibromyalgia symptoms. Foods that support gut health include those high in fiber, like fruits, vegetables, and whole grains, as well as fermented foods such as yogurt, kefir, and sauerkraut, which introduce beneficial probiotics into the digestive system.

Blood sugar regulation is important for maintaining energy levels and reducing fatigue. Foods with a high glycemic index, such as white bread, pastries, and sugary drinks, can cause rapid spikes and drops in blood sugar levels, leading to energy crashes and increased fatigue. In contrast, complex carbohydrates found in whole grains, legumes, and vegetables provide a more stable release of energy, helping to maintain steady blood sugar levels and reduce fatigue.

Neurotransmitter function is also influenced by diet. Neurotransmitters like serotonin and dopamine, which play roles in mood regulation and pain perception, are affected by the nutrients we consume. For example, tryptophan, an amino acid found in turkey, eggs, and nuts, is a precursor to serotonin. Ensuring adequate intake of such nutrients can support neurotransmitter function, potentially improving mood and reducing pain perception in fibromyalgia patients.

Additionally, **magnesium deficiency** has been linked to increased pain and fatigue in fibromyalgia. Magnesium plays a crucial role in muscle function and energy production. Foods rich in magnesium, such as spinach, almonds, and avocados, can help address this deficiency and improve symptoms.

By understanding the scientific explanations behind these dietary impacts, individuals with fibromyalgia can better manage their symptoms through targeted nutritional strategies. This strategy offers a complete way to enhance the quality of life for fibromyalgia sufferers by supporting general health and well-being in addition to reducing pain and inflammation.

Conclusion

Nutrition plays a vital role in managing fibromyalgia, a condition characterized by widespread pain and fatigue. While there's no one-size-fits-all diet, understanding how food affects symptoms can significantly improve quality of life. Avoiding processed foods, sugars, and additives helps prevent flare-ups, while a diet rich in fruits, vegetables, lean proteins, and healthy fats supports recovery and boosts energy.

Recognizing how these foods affect inflammation, oxidative stress, gut health, blood sugar, and nutrient levels can guide better dietary choices. By focusing on anti-inflammatory and nutrient-dense foods, individuals can manage pain and fatigue more effectively. Consistent application of these nutritional strategies can lead to better symptom control and an enhanced quality of life for those with fibromyalgia.

CHAPTER 6: 5-WEEK MEAL PLAN

Embarking on a new dietary plan can seem daunting, especially when dealing with a chronic condition like fibromyalgia. However, the 5-week meal plan outlined in this chapter is designed to be a practical and effective way to manage symptoms and improve overall health. Each week builds on the previous one, guiding you through a structured approach to detoxify, reduce inflammation, boost energy, improve digestion, and maintain a balanced diet. While the plan might seem repetitive or tedious at times, sticking with it is crucial for long-term benefits. Patience and consistency are key to experiencing the full advantages of these dietary changes.

This meal plan focuses on incorporating whole foods that are rich in essential nutrients. Every week's foundation is made up of whole grains, lean meats, fresh produce, and healthy fats. These foods are not only nutritious but also help reduce inflammation and support overall well-being. By eliminating processed foods and introducing anti-inflammatory ingredients, you'll begin to notice improvements in your energy levels and symptom management.

It's important to recognize that achieving optimal nutrition can sometimes be challenging, especially if you have specific dietary restrictions or preferences. If you find it difficult to get all the necessary nutrients from food alone, consider incorporating dietary supplements. For example, omega-3 supplements can help reduce inflammation, while probiotics support gut health. Vitamin D and magnesium supplements can also be beneficial, particularly for individuals with fibromyalgia who may have deficiencies in these areas.

Remember, this plan is not just about what you eat, but also about fostering a healthier relationship with food. Take the time to plan, prepare, and enjoy your meals. Your commitment to this 5-week meal plan can lead to significant improvements in your health and quality of life.

WEEK 1: DETOX AND CLEANSE

The first week of our 5-week meal plan focuses on detoxification and cleansing. This initial phase aims to reset your body by eliminating processed foods and introducing anti-inflammatory ingredients. The goal is to remove toxins that can contribute to inflammation and exacerbate fibromyalgia symptoms, setting a solid foundation for the weeks ahead.

Start by **eliminating processed foods**. These foods are often high in unhealthy fats, sugars, and artificial additives that can increase inflammation and stress your body. Processed snacks, fast foods, sugary beverages, and pre-packaged meals should be avoided. Instead, focus on whole, natural foods that provide essential nutrients without the harmful additives. Fresh fruits, vegetables, lean proteins, and whole grains will be your staples this week.

Incorporate **anti-inflammatory ingredients** into your meals. Foods rich in antioxidants, vitamins, and minerals can help reduce inflammation and support your body's natural detox processes. Leafy greens like spinach and kale, colorful vegetables like bell peppers and carrots, and fruits such as berries and oranges are excellent choices. These foods not only help cleanse your system but also provide a burst of nutrients that promote overall health.

Hydration is another crucial element of detoxification. Drinking plenty of water helps flush out toxins and keeps your body functioning optimally. Aim for at least eight glasses of water a day. Herbal teas, such as green tea or chamomile, can also support detox efforts with their natural antioxidant properties.

To support your detox, consider starting your day with a **nutritious smoothie**. Blend spinach, kale, a banana, some berries, and a splash of almond milk for a delicious and detoxifying start to your morning. Adding a tablespoon of chia seeds or flaxseeds can boost fiber intake, aiding in digestion and further promoting detoxification.

Mindful eating practices can enhance the detox process. Take your time to eat, savor each bite, and listen to your body's hunger and fullness cues. This can help improve digestion and ensure you are getting the most out of the nutritious foods you are consuming.

By the end of the first week, you should feel a noticeable difference in your energy levels and overall well-being. Eliminating processed foods and embracing anti-inflammatory ingredients lays a strong foundation for the subsequent phases of this meal plan. This detox and cleanse phase is not just about removing toxins but also about nourishing your body with the nutrients it needs to thrive.

WEEK 2: REDUCING INFLAMMATION

The second week of the 5-week meal plan focuses on reducing inflammation by incorporating foods rich in antioxidants and omega-3 fatty acids. These nutrients play a crucial role in fighting inflammation and alleviating the pain and discomfort associated with fibromyalgia.

Start by **adding more antioxidants** to your diet. Antioxidants help neutralize free radicals in the body, which can cause cellular damage and increase inflammation. Foods rich in antioxidants include berries such as blueberries, strawberries, and raspberries. These fruits are not only delicious but also packed with vitamins and fiber. Leafy greens like spinach, kale, and Swiss chard are also excellent sources of antioxidants, as well as vitamins A, C, and K.

Omega-3 fatty acids are essential for reducing inflammation and supporting overall health. Fatty fish like salmon, mackerel, and sardines are some of the best sources of omega-3s. If you're not a fan of fish, consider incorporating plant-based sources like chia seeds, flaxseeds, and walnuts into your meals. These can be easily added to smoothies, salads, and oatmeal.

Nuts and seeds are another great addition to your anti-inflammatory diet. Almonds, walnuts, and sunflower seeds are not only rich in omega-3s but also provide a good dose of antioxidants and healthy fats. Snacking on a handful of nuts or adding them to your dishes can be a simple yet effective way to boost your intake of these nutrients.

Herbs and spices can also help reduce inflammation. Turmeric, with its active compound curcumin, is renowned for its anti-inflammatory properties. Adding a pinch of turmeric to your meals, such as soups, stews, or even smoothies, can provide significant benefits. Ginger, garlic, and cinnamon are other spices known for their anti-inflammatory effects and can be easily incorporated into various dishes.

Incorporating these foods into your daily meals doesn't have to be complicated. Start your day with a smoothie packed with spinach, berries, and a tablespoon of chia seeds. For lunch, enjoy a salad topped with walnuts, avocado, and a simple olive oil and lemon dressing. Dinner could feature a serving of grilled salmon with a side of steamed vegetables and quinoa.

By the end of this week, you should notice a reduction in inflammation and an improvement in your overall well-being. This focus on antioxidant-rich foods and omega-3 fatty acids not only helps manage fibromyalgia symptoms but also supports your overall health.

WEEK 3: BOOSTING ENERGY

The third week of our 5-week meal plan is dedicated to boosting energy levels. For individuals with fibromyalgia, fatigue can be one of the most debilitating symptoms. By incorporating nutrient-dense superfoods into your diet, you can enhance your energy and overall vitality.

Nutrient-dense superfoods are packed with vitamins, minerals, and antioxidants that provide sustained energy throughout the day. Start by incorporating more **leafy greens** like kale, spinach, and Swiss chard. These vegetables are rich in iron, which is crucial for energy production, as well as magnesium, which supports muscle and nerve function.

Berries such as blueberries, strawberries, and raspberries are another excellent addition. They are high in antioxidants and vitamin C, which can help reduce oxidative stress and boost your immune system. Adding a handful of berries to your breakfast or as a snack can provide a quick and nutritious energy boost.

Whole grains are essential for maintaining steady energy levels. High in fiber and complex carbs, foods like quinoa, brown rice, oats, and barley help control blood sugar levels and ward off energy slumps. Starting your day with a bowl of oatmeal topped with fresh fruit and nuts is a great way to fuel your body.

Nuts and seeds such as almonds, walnuts, chia seeds, and flaxseeds are rich in healthy fats, protein, and fiber. These superfoods provide a slow release of energy and keep you feeling full longer. They are also easy to incorporate into meals and snacks. Try adding chia seeds to your smoothie or sprinkling flaxseeds on your salad for an extra nutritional punch.

Lean proteins are vital for muscle repair and energy. Incorporate sources like chicken, turkey, tofu, and legumes into your diet. Proteins help maintain muscle mass and support metabolic functions, which are essential for sustained energy. A lunch featuring grilled chicken breast with a quinoa and vegetable salad can be both satisfying and energizing.

Hydration is equally important for maintaining energy levels. Dehydration can lead to fatigue and decreased cognitive function. Aim to drink plenty of water throughout the day, and include hydrating foods like cucumbers, oranges, and watermelon.

Finally, consider incorporating **adaptogenic herbs** like ashwagandha and ginseng. These herbs are known for their energy-boosting properties and can help your body adapt to stress. They can be found in teas, supplements, or added to smoothies.

By the end of this week, you should notice a significant improvement in your energy levels. Integrating these nutrient-dense superfoods into your daily meals provides your body with the essential nutrients it needs to function optimally, helping to combat fatigue and enhance your overall well-being.

WEEK 4: IMPROVING DIGESTION

The fourth week of our 5-week meal plan is dedicated to improving digestion. For those with fibromyalgia, digestive issues are common and can exacerbate symptoms like pain and fatigue. Focusing on gut health with probiotics and fiber-rich foods can significantly enhance your digestive system's efficiency and overall well-being.

Start by incorporating **probiotics** into your diet. Probiotics are beneficial bacteria that support a healthy gut microbiome. They can be found in fermented foods such as yogurt, kefir, sauerkraut, kimchi, and miso. These foods help balance the gut flora, improving digestion and boosting the immune system. A daily serving of probiotic-rich yogurt or a spoonful of sauerkraut can make a big difference in gut health.

Fiber-rich foods are essential for maintaining regular bowel movements and preventing constipation, a common issue for many with fibromyalgia. Foods high in fiber include whole grains, fruits, vegetables, legumes, and seeds. Soluble fiber, found in oats, apples, and beans, helps regulate blood sugar levels and supports heart health. Insoluble fiber, found in whole wheat, nuts, and many vegetables, adds bulk to the stool and aids in its passage through the digestive tract. Aim to include a variety of these fiber sources in your daily meals.

Hydration plays a crucial role in digestion. Water helps dissolve nutrients and waste products, making it easier for them to pass through the digestive system. Drinking plenty of water throughout the day helps prevent dehydration and supports digestive health. Herbal teas, such as peppermint and ginger tea, can also soothe the digestive tract and reduce symptoms like bloating and gas.

Incorporate digestive enzymes to aid in the breakdown of food and enhance nutrient absorption. Pineapple and papaya are natural sources of digestive enzymes like bromelain and papain. Adding these fruits to your diet can help improve digestion, especially after heavy meals.

Mindful eating practices can further enhance digestion. Eating slowly, chewing food thoroughly, and paying attention to your body's hunger and fullness cues can prevent overeating and reduce digestive discomfort. Avoiding distractions like television or work during meals allows you to focus on your food and enjoy the process of eating.

By the end of this week, you should experience improved digestion and a reduction in gastrointestinal discomfort. A focus on probiotics, fiber-rich foods, and proper hydration supports a healthy gut, which is essential for overall health and can help alleviate some of the symptoms associated with fibromyalgia. Integrating these practices into your routine sets the stage for long-term digestive health and well-being.

WEEK 5: MAINTENANCE AND STABILITY

The final week of the 5-week meal plan focuses on maintaining a balanced diet for long-term health. After detoxing, reducing inflammation, boosting energy, and improving digestion, it's essential to establish a sustainable eating pattern that supports ongoing wellness and symptom management.

A **balanced diet** incorporates a variety of food groups in appropriate proportions. This entails keeping whole foods—such as fruits, vegetables, whole grains, lean meats, and healthy fats—as the top priority. Variety is key to ensuring you receive a wide range of nutrients necessary for optimal health.

Meal planning and preparation become crucial in this phase. Take time each week to plan your meals, ensuring they include a balance of macronutrients and are rich in vitamins and minerals. Preparing meals in advance can help you avoid the temptation of processed and convenience foods, which can trigger fibromyalgia symptoms.

Consistency in eating habits is also important. Try to maintain regular meal times and avoid skipping meals, which can lead to energy crashes and increased pain. Balanced snacks between meals, such as a handful of nuts or a piece of fruit, can help keep your energy levels stable throughout the day.

Listen to your body and adjust your diet as needed. Everyone's experience with fibromyalgia is unique, and dietary needs can change over time. Pay attention to how different foods affect your symptoms and be willing to make adjustments. Keeping a food journal can help you track what works best for you.

Incorporate mindfulness into your eating habits. Eating slowly and savoring your food can improve digestion and help you enjoy your meals more fully. In addition, it enables you to pay attention to your body's signals of hunger and fullness, which helps you avoid overindulging and advance your health.

Stay hydrated by drinking plenty of water throughout the day. Proper hydration supports all bodily functions and can help reduce fatigue and improve cognitive function. Herbal teas and water-rich foods like cucumbers and melons can also contribute to your daily hydration needs.

Physical activity complements a balanced diet. Regular exercise can help manage fibromyalgia symptoms, improve mood, and boost overall health. Choose activities you enjoy and can sustain long-term, such as walking, swimming, or yoga.

By the end of this week, you should have established a balanced and sustainable eating pattern that supports your long-term health. This phase is about finding stability and making your new dietary habits a permanent part of your lifestyle. Maintaining a balanced diet not only helps manage fibromyalgia symptoms but also enhances overall well-being, enabling you to live a healthier, more fulfilling life.

Conclusion

Completing the 5-week meal plan is a significant achievement and a testament to your commitment to improving your health. By following this structured approach, you have taken proactive steps to manage your fibromyalgia symptoms through better nutrition. Each week, from detoxifying your body to maintaining a balanced diet, has provided you with the tools and knowledge needed to sustain these healthy habits long-term.

It's important to acknowledge that sticking to this plan may have been challenging at times. Repetition and routine can feel monotonous, but consistency is essential for seeing results. Patience is crucial as your body adjusts to these dietary changes. The benefits of reduced inflammation, increased energy levels, improved digestion, and overall enhanced well-being are well worth the effort.

If you find that you're still struggling to meet your nutritional needs, don't hesitate to incorporate supplements into your diet. Omega-3 supplements, for instance, can further aid in reducing inflammation. Probiotics can bolster your gut health, while vitamin D and magnesium supplements can address common deficiencies. These additions can complement your diet and ensure you receive the full spectrum of necessary nutrients.

As you move forward, continue to prioritize whole, nutrient-dense foods. Keep experimenting with new recipes and flavors to keep your meals exciting and enjoyable. Remember, the habits you've developed over these five weeks are building blocks for a healthier future. Maintaining these dietary practices will help you manage your fibromyalgia symptoms more effectively and enhance your overall quality of life.

Stay committed to your health journey, and don't be discouraged by setbacks. Every small step you take towards better nutrition is a step towards a healthier, more vibrant life.

CHAPTER 7: RECIPES FOR FIBROMYALGIA

In this chapter, you will embark on a journey through a world of nutritional delights. Each recipe combines unique flavors and delicious ingredients to offer a variety of options aimed at combating the symptoms of fibromyalgia and reducing inflammation. By focusing on nutrient-dense, anti-inflammatory foods, these recipes are designed to support your body in its healing process.

Switching to a diet that eliminates processed foods and dairy products may seem daunting at first, but the benefits for your health are profound. Processed foods and dairy can often contribute to inflammation and exacerbate symptoms of fibromyalgia. By choosing whole, natural ingredients, you provide your body with the essential nutrients it needs to function optimally and reduce inflammation.

Embrace the change with enthusiasm and patience. Each meal you prepare from these recipes is a step towards a healthier, more vibrant you. The delicious flavors and satisfying dishes will make the transition smoother, ensuring that you don't feel deprived but rather empowered by the positive changes you're making for your health.

BREAKFAST

RECIPE 1: TOAST WITH AVOCADO AND POACHED EGG

Prep Time: 10 minutes
Servings: 1
Cooking Method: Stovetop
Nutritional Values:

- Calories: 250
- Protein: 10g
- Carbohydrates: 20g
- Fat: 15g

Difficulty: 2/5

Ingredients:

- 1 slice whole grain bread
- 1/2 ripe avocado
- 1 large egg
- 1 tsp lemon juice
- Salt and pepper to taste
- Pinch of red pepper flakes (optional)

Procedure:

- Toast the whole grain bread to your desired crispness.
- Mash the avocado in a small bowl and mix with lemon juice, salt, and pepper.
- Spread the avocado mixture onto the toasted bread.
- Bring a small pot of water to a gentle simmer. Crack the egg into a small bowl and gently slide it into the water. Poach for about 3 minutes.
- Remove the egg with a slotted spoon and place it on top of the avocado toast.
- Sprinkle with red pepper flakes if desired.

RECIPE 2: ANTI-INFLAMMATORY SMOOTHIE BOWL

Prep Time: 5 minutes
Servings: 1
Cooking Method: Blender
Nutritional Values:

- Calories: 350
- Protein: 8g
- Carbohydrates: 45g
- Fat: 15g

Difficulty: 1/5

Ingredients:

- 1/2 cup frozen blueberries
- 1/2 cup frozen spinach
- 1 banana
- 1/2 cup almond milk
- 1 tbsp chia seeds
- 1 tbsp almond butter
- Toppings: sliced banana, fresh berries, granola

Procedure:

- Combine blueberries, spinach, banana, almond milk, chia seeds, and almond butter in a blender.
- Blend until smooth and thick.
- Pour into a bowl and top with sliced banana, fresh berries, and granola.

RECIPE 3: ALMOND FLOUR PANCAKES

Prep Time: 15 minutes
Servings: 1
Cooking Method: Stovetop
Nutritional Values:

- Calories: 400
- Protein: 14g
- Carbohydrates: 12g
- Fat: 34g

Difficulty: 2/5

Ingredients:

- 1 cup almond flour
- 2 large eggs
- 1/4 cup unsweetened almond milk
- 1 tbsp maple syrup
- 1 tsp baking powder
- 1/4 tsp salt
- 1 tsp vanilla extract
- Coconut oil for cooking

Procedure:

- Combine almond flour, baking powder, and salt in a bowl.
- Combine the wet and dry ingredients until smooth.
- Heat a non-stick skillet over medium heat and grease with coconut oil.
- Pour batter into the skillet to form small pancakes. Cook for 2-3 minutes on each side until golden brown.

RECIPE 4: CHIA SEED PUDDING

Prep Time: 10 minutes + overnight chilling
Servings: 1
Cooking Method: No-cook
Nutritional Values:

- Calories: 300
- Protein: 6g
- Carbohydrates: 20g
- Fat: 20g

Difficulty: 1/5

Ingredients:

- 1/4 cup chia seeds
- 1 cup coconut milk
- 1 tbsp maple syrup
- 1/2 tsp vanilla extract
- Fresh berries for topping

Procedure:

- In a jar, combine chia seeds, coconut milk, maple syrup, and vanilla extract.
- Stir well to combine.
- Refrigerate overnight or for at least 4 hours.
- Stir before serving and top with fresh berries.

RECIPE 5: QUINOA BREAKFAST BOWL

Prep Time: 20 minutes
Servings: 1
Cooking Method: Stovetop
Nutritional Values:

- Calories: 350
- Protein: 9g
- Carbohydrates: 60g
- Fat: 10g

Difficulty: 2/5

Ingredients:

- 1/2 cup cooked quinoa
- 1/2 cup almond milk
- 1 tbsp almond butter
- 1 banana, sliced
- 1/4 cup blueberries
- 1 tbsp honey
- 1/4 tsp cinnamon

Procedure:

- In a small pot, heat the cooked quinoa and almond milk over medium heat until warm.
- Stir in almond butter and cinnamon.
- Transfer to a bowl and top with sliced banana, blueberries, and a drizzle of honey.

RECIPE 6: SPINACH AND MUSHROOM OMELET

Prep Time: 10 minutes
Servings: 1
Cooking Method: Stovetop
Nutritional Values:
Calories: 200
Protein: 14g
Carbohydrates: 3g
Fat: 15g
Difficulty: 2/5

Ingredients:

- 2 large eggs
- 1/4 cup chopped spinach
- 1/4 cup sliced mushrooms
- 1 tbsp olive oil
- Salt and pepper to taste

Procedure:

- Beat the eggs in a bowl and season with salt and pepper.
- Heat olive oil in a non-stick skillet over medium heat.
- Add mushrooms and spinach, cooking until soft.
- Pour in the eggs and cook until the edges start to set.
- Fold the omelet in half and cook until fully set.

RECIPE 7: BLUEBERRY OATMEAL

Prep Time: 10 minutes
Servings: 1
Cooking Method: Stovetop
Nutritional Values:

- Calories: 250
- Protein: 6g
- Carbohydrates: 50g
- Fat: 5g

Difficulty: 1/5

Ingredients:

- 1/2 cup rolled oats
- 1 cup water or almond milk
- 1/2 cup blueberries
- 1 tbsp chia seeds
- 1 tbsp honey
- 1/4 tsp cinnamon

Procedure:

- In a pot, bring water or almond milk to a boil.
- Add rolled oats and reduce heat to a simmer.
- Cook until oats are tender, about 5 minutes.
- Stir in blueberries, chia seeds, honey, and cinnamon.
- Serve warm.

RECIPE 8: GREEK YOGURT WITH HONEY AND NUTS

Prep Time: 5 minutes
Servings: 1
Cooking Method: No-cook
Nutritional Values:

- Calories: 300
- Protein: 18g
- Carbohydrates: 30g
- Fat: 12g

Difficulty: 1/5

Ingredients:

- 1 cup Greek yogurt
- 1 tbsp honey
- 2 tbsp chopped walnuts
- 1 tbsp chia seeds

Procedure:

- Place Greek yogurt in a bowl.
- Drizzle with honey and sprinkle with chopped walnuts and chia seeds.
- Mix well and serve.

RECIPE 9: SWEET POTATO AND BLACK BEAN HASH

Prep Time: 20 minutes
Servings: 1
Cooking Method: Stovetop
Nutritional Values:

- Calories: 300
- Protein: 8g
- Carbohydrates: 50g
- Fat: 10g

Difficulty: 2/5

Ingredients:

- 1 small sweet potato, diced
- 1/2 cup black beans, drained and rinsed
- 1/4 cup diced bell pepper
- 1/4 cup diced onion
- 1 tbsp olive oil
- Salt and pepper to taste

Procedure:

- Heat olive oil in a skillet over medium heat.
- Add diced sweet potato and cook until tender, about 10 minutes.
- Add bell pepper, onion, and black beans. Cook until vegetables are soft.
- Season with salt and pepper.

Prep Time: 15 minutes
Servings: 1
Cooking Method: Stovetop
Nutritional Values:

- Calories: 350
- Protein: 20g
- Carbohydrates: 30g
- Fat: 15g

Difficulty: 2/5

Ingredients:

- 1 ripe banana
- 2 large eggs
- 1/4 cup protein powder (vanilla flavor)
- 1/4 tsp baking powder
- 1/4 tsp cinnamon
- Coconut oil for cooking

Procedure:

- In a bowl, mash the banana until smooth.
- Add eggs, protein powder, baking powder, and cinnamon. Mix well.
- Heat a non-stick skillet over medium heat and grease with coconut oil.
- Pour batter into the skillet to form small pancakes. Cook for 2-3 minutes on each side until golden brown.

RECIPE 11: QUINOA AND VEGETABLE SALAD

Prep Time: 20 minutes
Servings: 1
Cooking Method: No-cook
Nutritional Values:

- Calories: 300
- Protein: 8g
- Carbohydrates: 35g
- Fat: 14g

Difficulty: 1/5

Ingredients:

- 1/2 cup cooked quinoa
- 1/4 cup diced cucumber
- 1/4 cup cherry tomatoes, halved
- 1/4 cup chopped bell pepper
- 1/4 cup diced red onion
- 2 tbsp chopped fresh parsley
- 1 tbsp olive oil
- 1 tbsp lemon juice
- Salt and pepper to taste

Procedure:

- Put the cooked quinoa, cucumber, cherry tomatoes, red onion, bell pepper, and parsley in a big bowl.
- Mix the olive oil, lemon juice, salt, and pepper in a small bowl.
- Drizzle the quinoa mixture with the dressing, tossing to blend.
- Serve chilled or at room temperature.

RECIPE 12: RED LENTIL SOUP

Prep Time: 30 minutes
Servings: 1
Cooking Method: Stovetop
Nutritional Values:

- Calories: 250
- Protein: 14g
- Carbohydrates: 40g
- Fat: 6g

Difficulty: 2/5

Ingredients:

- 1/2 cup red lentils, rinsed
- 1 small carrot, diced
- 1 small onion, diced
- 1 celery stalk, diced
- 2 cups vegetable broth
- 1 garlic clove, minced
- 1 tsp ground cumin
- 1 tsp turmeric
- 1 tbsp olive oil
- Salt and pepper to taste

Procedure:

- In a pot over medium heat, warm the olive oil. Add the celery, carrot, onion, and garlic, and sauté the veggies until they are tender.
- After adding the turmeric and cumin, stir for one minute.

- Include the veggie broth and lentils. Once the lentils are soft, bring to a boil, then lower the heat and simmer for 20 minutes.
- Add pepper and salt for seasoning.
- If preferred, mix the soup with an immersion blender until it's smooth.

RECIPE 13: CHICKEN AND AVOCADO WRAP

Prep Time: 15 minutes
Servings: 1
Cooking Method: No-cook
Nutritional Values:

- Calories: 350
- Protein: 25g
- Carbohydrates: 30g
- Fat: 14g

Difficulty: 1/5

Ingredients:

- 1 whole wheat tortilla
- 1/2 cooked chicken breast, sliced
- 1/2 avocado, sliced
- 1/4 cup shredded lettuce
- 1/4 cup shredded carrot
- 1 tbsp Greek yogurt
- 1 tsp lemon juice
- Salt and pepper to taste

Procedure:

- In a small bowl, mix Greek yogurt, lemon juice, salt, and pepper.
- Lay the tortilla flat and spread the yogurt mixture evenly over it.
- Arrange chicken, avocado, lettuce, and carrot on top.
- Roll up the tortilla tightly and cut in half.

RECIPE 14: MEDITERRANEAN CHICKPEA SALAD

Prep Time: 10 minutes
Servings: 1
Cooking Method: No-cook
Nutritional Values:

- Calories: 300
- Protein: 10g
- Carbohydrates: 28g
- Fat: 16g

Difficulty: 1/5

Ingredients:

- 1/2 cup canned chickpeas, rinsed and drained
- 1/4 cup diced cucumber
- 1/4 cup cherry tomatoes, halved
- 1/4 cup diced red onion
- 2 tbsp crumbled feta cheese
- 1 tbsp olive oil
- 1 tbsp red wine vinegar
- 1 tsp dried oregano
- Salt and pepper to taste

Procedure:

- Combine the feta cheese, tomatoes, cucumber, red onion, and chickpeas in a sizable bowl.

- Combine the olive oil, red wine vinegar, oregano, salt, and pepper in a small bowl.
- Combine the olive oil, red wine vinegar, oregano, salt, and pepper in a small bowl.
- Serve chilled or at room temperature.

RECIPE 15: GRILLED VEGETABLE PANINI

Prep Time: 15 minutes
Servings: 1
Cooking Method: Stovetop or Panini press
Nutritional Values:

- Calories: 350
- Protein: 12g
- Carbohydrates: 40g
- Fat: 16g

Difficulty: 2/5

Ingredients:

- 2 slices whole grain bread
- 1/4 cup sliced zucchini
- 1/4 cup sliced bell pepper
- 1/4 cup sliced eggplant
- 1 tbsp olive oil
- 1 tbsp pesto sauce
- 1 slice provolone cheese
- Salt and pepper to taste

Procedure:

- Slices of bell pepper, eggplant, and zucchini should be brushed with olive oil and seasoned with salt and pepper.
- Grill the vegetables on a stovetop grill pan or Panini press until tender.
- Spread pesto sauce on one side of each bread slice.
- Layer the grilled vegetables and provolone cheese between the bread slices.
- Grill the sandwich in a Panini press or on a stovetop grill pan until the bread is toasted and the cheese is melted.

RECIPE 16: SPINACH AND FETA STUFFED PEPPERS

Prep Time: 30 minutes
Servings: 1
Cooking Method: Oven
Nutritional Values:

- Calories: 250
- Protein: 8g
- Carbohydrates: 30g
- Fat: 12g

Difficulty: 3/5

Ingredients:

- 1 bell pepper, halved and seeds removed
- 1/2 cup cooked quinoa
- 1/4 cup chopped spinach
- 2 tbsp crumbled feta cheese
- 1 garlic clove, minced
- 1 tbsp olive oil
- Salt and pepper to taste

Procedure:

- Preheat oven to 375°F (190°C).
- In a bowl, combine cooked quinoa, spinach, feta cheese, garlic, olive oil, salt, and pepper.
- Stuff the mixture into the bell pepper halves.
- Place the stuffed peppers on a baking sheet and bake for 20-25 minutes, or until the peppers are tender.

RECIPE 17: SALMON AND AVOCADO SALAD

Prep Time: 20 minutes
Servings: 1
Cooking Method: No-cook (if using pre-cooked salmon)
Nutritional Values:

- Calories: 350
- Protein: 20g
- Carbohydrates: 15g
- Fat: 25g

Difficulty: 1/5

Ingredients:

- 3 oz cooked salmon, flaked
- 1/2 avocado, sliced
- 1 cup mixed greens
- 1/4 cup cherry tomatoes, halved
- 1 tbsp olive oil
- 1 tbsp lemon juice
- Salt and pepper to taste

Procedure:

- In a large bowl, combine mixed greens, cherry tomatoes, salmon, and avocado.
- In a small bowl, whisk together olive oil, lemon juice, salt, and pepper.
- Drizzle the dressing over the salad and toss gently to combine.
- Serve immediately.

RECIPE 18: QUINOA AND ROASTED VEGETABLE SALAD

Prep Time: 30 minutes
Servings: 1
Cooking Method: Oven
Nutritional Values:

- Calories: 350
- Protein: 10g
- Carbohydrates: 50g
- Fat: 14g

Difficulty: 2/5

Ingredients:

- 1/2 cup quinoa, cooked
- 1/2 cup cherry tomatoes, halved
- 1/2 cup zucchini, diced
- 1/2 cup bell pepper, diced
- 1/4 cup red onion, diced
- 1 tbsp olive oil
- 1 tbsp balsamic vinegar
- 1 tsp dried oregano
- Salt and pepper to taste

Procedure:

- Preheat oven to 400°F (200°C).
- Toss the cherry tomatoes, zucchini, bell pepper, and red onion with olive oil, salt, and pepper.
- Spread the vegetables on a baking sheet and roast for 20 minutes.
- In a large bowl, combine the cooked quinoa, roasted vegetables, balsamic vinegar, and dried oregano.
- Mix well and serve warm or chilled.

RECIPE 19: LENTIL AND SPINACH WRAP

Prep Time: 20 minutes
Servings: 1
Cooking Method: No-cook
Nutritional Values:

- Calories: 320
- Protein: 14g
- Carbohydrates: 50g
- Fat: 8g

Difficulty: 1/5
Procedure:

Ingredients:

- 1/2 cup cooked lentils
- 1 cup fresh spinach
- 1/4 cup diced cucumber
- 1/4 cup shredded carrot
- 1 whole wheat tortilla
- 2 tbsp hummus
- Salt and pepper to taste

- Spread hummus evenly over the tortilla.
- Layer the cooked lentils, spinach, cucumber, and carrot on the tortilla.
- Season with salt and pepper.
- Roll the tortilla tightly and cut in half.

RECIPE 20: TURKEY AND AVOCADO SALAD

Prep Time: 15 minutes
Servings: 1
Cooking Method: No-cook
Nutritional Values:

- Calories: 350
- Protein: 20g
- Carbohydrates: 15g
- Fat: 25g

Difficulty: 1/5

Ingredients:

- 3 oz cooked turkey breast, sliced
- 1/2 avocado, diced
- 2 cups mixed greens
- 1/4 cup cherry tomatoes, halved
- 1/4 cup diced cucumber
- 1 tbsp olive oil
- 1 tbsp apple cider vinegar
- Salt and pepper to taste

Procedure:

- In a large bowl, combine mixed greens, cherry tomatoes, cucumber, turkey, and avocado.
- In a small bowl, whisk together olive oil, apple cider vinegar, salt, and pepper.
- Pour the dressing over the salad and toss gently to combine.
- Serve immediately.

RECIPE 21: SPINACH AND FETA QUINOA BOWL

Prep Time: 20 minutes
Servings: 1
Cooking Method: No-cook
Nutritional Values:

- Calories: 350
- Protein: 12g
- Carbohydrates: 35g
- Fat: 18g

Difficulty: 1/5

Ingredients:

- 1/2 cup cooked quinoa
- 1 cup fresh spinach
- 1/4 cup crumbled feta cheese
- 1/4 cup cherry tomatoes, halved
- 1/4 cup diced cucumber
- 1 tbsp olive oil
- 1 tbsp lemon juice
- Salt and pepper to taste

Procedure:

- In a large bowl, combine quinoa, spinach, feta cheese, cherry tomatoes, and cucumber.
- In a small bowl, whisk together olive oil, lemon juice, salt, and pepper.
- Pour the dressing over the quinoa mixture and toss to combine.
- Serve immediately.

RECIPE 22: SALAD WITH BLACK BEAN AND CORN

Prep Time: 15 minutes
Servings: 1
Cooking Method: No-cook
Nutritional Values:

- Calories: 250
- Protein: 8g
- Carbohydrates: 40g
- Fat: 8g

Difficulty: 1/5

Ingredients:

- 1/2 cup canned black beans, rinsed and drained
- 1/2 cup canned corn, rinsed and drained
- 1/4 cup diced red bell pepper
- 1/4 cup diced red onion
- 1 tbsp chopped fresh cilantro
- 1 tbsp olive oil
- 1 tbsp lime juice

- Salt and pepper to taste

Procedure:

- In a large bowl, combine black beans, corn, bell pepper, red onion, and cilantro.
- In a small bowl, whisk together olive oil, lime juice, salt, and pepper.
- Pour the dressing over the bean mixture and toss to combine.
- Serve immediately or chilled.

RECIPE 23: GRILLED CHICKEN AND VEGGIE SKEWERS

Prep Time: 30 minutes
Servings: 1
Cooking Method: Grill
Nutritional Values:

- Calories: 300
- Protein: 25g
- Carbohydrates: 10g
- Fat: 15g

Difficulty: 2/5

Ingredients:

- 4 oz chicken breast, cubed
- 1/4 cup bell pepper, cubed
- 1/4 cup zucchini, sliced
- 1/4 cup cherry tomatoes
- 1 tbsp olive oil
- 1 tbsp lemon juice
- 1 tsp dried oregano
- Salt and pepper to taste

Procedure:

- Preheat the grill to medium-high heat.
- In a bowl, combine chicken, bell pepper, zucchini, and cherry tomatoes.
- In a small bowl, whisk together olive oil, lemon juice, oregano, salt, and pepper.
- Pour the marinade over the chicken and vegetables, tossing to coat.
- Thread the chicken and vegetables onto skewers.
- Grill the skewers for 10-12 minutes, turning occasionally, until the chicken is cooked through.

RECIPE 24: VEGGIE AND HUMMUS SANDWICH

Prep Time: 10 minutes
Servings: 1
Cooking Method: No-cook
Nutritional Values:

- Calories: 300
- Protein: 10g
- Carbohydrates: 45g

Ingredients:

- 2 slices whole grain bread
- 3 tbsp hummus
- 1/4 cup shredded carrot
- 1/4 cup sliced cucumber
- 1/4 cup sliced bell pepper
- Handful of spinach leaves

- Fat: 10g
- Salt and pepper to taste

Difficulty: 1/5

Procedure:

- Spread hummus evenly over one side of each bread slice.
- Layer the carrot, cucumber, bell pepper, and spinach leaves on one slice of bread.
- Season with salt and pepper.
- Top with the other slice of bread and cut in half.

RECIPE 25: TOFU AND VEGGIE STIR-FRY

Prep Time: 20 minutes
Servings: 1
Cooking Method: Stovetop
Nutritional Values:

- Calories: 300
- Protein: 15g
- Carbohydrates: 25g
- Fat: 15g

Difficulty: 2/5

Ingredients:

- 4 oz firm tofu, cubed
- 1/2 cup broccoli florets
- 1/2 cup sliced bell pepper
- 1/4 cup sliced carrot
- 1 tbsp soy sauce
- 1 tbsp sesame oil
- 1 garlic clove, minced
- 1 tsp grated ginger
- 1 tsp sesame seeds
- Cooked brown rice (optional)

Procedure:

- Heat sesame oil in a large skillet over medium-high heat.
- Add garlic and ginger, and sauté for 1 minute.
- Add tofu, broccoli, bell pepper, and carrot. Stir-fry for 5-7 minutes.
- Add soy sauce and stir to combine.
- Sprinkle with sesame seeds before serving.
- Serve over cooked brown rice, if desired.

RECIPE 26: KALE AND SWEET POTATO SALAD

Prep Time: 30 minutes
Servings: 1
Cooking Method: Oven
Nutritional Values:

- Calories: 350
- Protein: 10g
- Carbohydrates: 40g
- Fat: 18g

Difficulty: 2/5

Ingredients:

- 1 cup chopped kale
- 1/2 small sweet potato, diced and roasted
- 1/4 cup cooked quinoa
- 1/4 cup diced apple
- 2 tbsp chopped walnuts
- 1 tbsp olive oil
- 1 tbsp apple cider vinegar
- 1 tsp honey
- Salt and pepper to taste

Procedure:

- Preheat oven to 400°F (200°C). Toss diced sweet potato with olive oil, salt, and pepper, and roast for 20 minutes.
- In a large bowl, combine kale, roasted sweet potato, quinoa, apple, and walnuts.
- In a small bowl, whisk together olive oil, apple cider vinegar, honey, salt, and pepper.
- Pour the dressing over the salad and toss to combine.
- Serve immediately or chilled.

RECIPE 27: QUINOA AND KALE SALAD

Prep Time: 20 minutes
Servings: 1
Cooking Method: Stovetop
Nutritional Values:

- Calories: 300
- Protein: 8g
- Carbs: 34g
- Fat: 16g

Difficulty: 2/5

Ingredients:

- 1/2 cup quinoa, rinsed
- 1 cup water
- 1 cup chopped kale
- 1/4 cup shredded carrots
- 1/4 cup chopped red bell pepper
- 1/4 cup diced cucumber
- 2 tbsp olive oil
- 1 tbsp lemon juice
- 1 tsp honey
- Salt and pepper to taste

Procedure:

- Quinoa and water should be combined in a small pot. After bringing to a boil, lower the heat, and simmer until the water is absorbed, about 15 minutes. Using a fork, fluff.

- Put the cooked quinoa, kale, carrots, bell pepper, and cucumber in a big bowl.
- Mix the olive oil, honey, lemon juice, salt, and pepper in a small bowl.
- Drizzle the salad with the dressing and toss to mix.

RECIPE 28: LENTIL AND SPINACH SOUP

Prep Time: 30 minutes
Servings: 1
Cooking Method: Stovetop
Nutritional Values:

- Calories: 250
- Protein: 14g
- Carbs: 38g
- Fat: 6g

Difficulty: 3/5

Ingredients:

- 1/2 cup dried lentils
- 2 cups vegetable broth
- 1/2 cup chopped spinach
- 1/4 cup diced tomatoes
- 1 small carrot, diced
- 1 small celery stalk, diced
- 1/2 small onion, diced
- 1 clove garlic, minced
- 1 tbsp olive oil
- Salt and pepper to taste

Procedure:

- Heat olive oil in a pot over medium heat. Add onion, garlic, carrot, and celery. Cook until softened, about 5 minutes.
- Add lentils and vegetable broth. Bring to a boil, then reduce heat and simmer for 20 minutes.
- Add spinach and tomatoes. Cook for another 5 minutes. Season with salt and pepper.

RECIPE 29: CHICKPEA AVOCADO WRAP

Prep Time: 15 minutes
Servings: 1
Cooking Method: None
Nutritional Values:

- Calories: 350
- Protein: 12g
- Carbs: 45g
- Fat: 15g

Difficulty: 1/5
Procedure:

Ingredients:

- 1/2 cup cooked chickpeas
- 1/2 avocado, mashed
- 1 tbsp lemon juice
- 1 tbsp chopped cilantro
- 1 whole wheat tortilla
- Salt and pepper to taste

- In a bowl, mash chickpeas with a fork. Add avocado, lemon juice, cilantro, salt, and pepper. Mix well.
- Spread the mixture onto the tortilla. Roll up and slice in half.

RECIPE 30: GRILLED CHICKEN AND VEGGIE BOWL

Prep Time: 25 minutes
Servings: 1
Cooking Method:
Grill/Stovetop
Nutritional Values:

- Calories: 400
- Protein: 30g
- Carbs: 50g
- Fat: 10g

Difficulty: 2/5

Ingredients:

- 1 small chicken breast, grilled and sliced
- 1/2 cup cooked brown rice
- 1/2 cup steamed broccoli
- 1/4 cup diced bell peppers
- 1/4 cup shredded carrots
- 2 tbsp teriyaki sauce

Procedure:

- Grill chicken breast until cooked through, about 5 minutes per side. Slice into strips.
- In a bowl, combine cooked brown rice, broccoli, bell peppers, and carrots.
- Top with sliced chicken and drizzle with teriyaki sauce.

RECIPE 31: TURKEY AND HUMMUS SANDWICH

Prep Time: 10 minutes
Servings: 1
Cooking Method: None
Nutritional Values:

- Calories: 350
- Protein: 25g
- Carbs: 40g
- Fat: 10g

Difficulty: 1/5

Ingredients:

- 2 slices whole grain bread
- 3 oz sliced turkey breast
- 2 tbsp hummus
- 1/4 cup baby spinach
- 1/4 cup sliced cucumbers

Procedure:

- Spread hummus on one slice of bread.
- Layer turkey, spinach, and cucumbers on top. Place the other slice of bread on top.
- Slice in half and serve.

RECIPE 32: SWEET POTATO AND BLACK BEAN SALAD

Prep Time: 30 minutes
Servings: 1
Cooking Method:
Oven/Stovetop
Nutritional Values:

- Calories: 300
- Protein: 10g
- Carbs: 50g
- Fat: 10g

Difficulty: 3/5

Ingredients:

- 1 small sweet potato, diced and roasted
- 1/2 cup black beans, rinsed and drained
- 1/4 cup diced red onion
- 1/4 cup chopped cilantro
- 1 tbsp olive oil
- 1 tbsp lime juice
- Salt and pepper to taste

Procedure:

- Preheat oven to 400°F. Toss sweet potato with a little olive oil, salt, and pepper. Roast for 20 minutes.
- In a bowl, combine roasted sweet potato, black beans, red onion, and cilantro.
- Drizzle with olive oil and lime juice. Toss to combine.

RECIPE 33: SPINACH AND FETA STUFFED PEPPERS

Prep Time: 40 minutes
Servings: 1
Cooking Method: Oven
Nutritional Values:

- Calories: 250
- Protein: 10g
- Carbs: 30g
- Fat: 12g

Difficulty: 3/5

Ingredients:

- 1 bell pepper, halved and seeded
- 1/2 cup cooked quinoa
- 1/4 cup crumbled feta cheese
- 1/4 cup chopped spinach
- 1 tbsp olive oil
- Salt and pepper to taste

Procedure:

- Preheat oven to 375°F. Place bell pepper halves on a baking sheet.
- In a bowl, mix quinoa, feta, spinach, olive oil, salt, and pepper.
- Stuff the pepper halves with the mixture. Bake for 25 minutes.

RECIPE 34: AVOCADO AND TUNA SALAD

Prep Time: 10 minutes
Servings: 1
Cooking Method: None
Nutritional Values:

- Calories: 300
- Protein: 25g
- Carbs: 10g
- Fat: 18g

Difficulty: 1/5

Ingredients:

- 1 can tuna in water, drained
- 1/2 avocado, diced
- 1 tbsp lemon juice
- 1 tbsp chopped parsley
- Salt and pepper to taste

Procedure:

- In a bowl, combine tuna, avocado, lemon juice, parsley, salt, and pepper.
- Mix well and serve on a bed of lettuce or whole grain toast.

RECIPE 35: ZUCCHINI NOODLES WITH PESTO

Prep Time: 15 minutes
Servings: 1
Cooking Method: Stovetop
Nutritional Values:
Calories: 200
Protein: 4g
Carbs: 12g
Fat: 18g
Difficulty: 2/5

Ingredients:

- 1 zucchini, spiralized
- 2 tbsp pesto sauce
- 1/4 cup cherry tomatoes, halved
- 1 tbsp pine nuts
- 1 tbsp olive oil
- Salt and pepper to taste

Procedure:

- Heat olive oil in a pan over medium heat. Add zucchini noodles and cook for 3-4 minutes.
- Add pesto sauce and cherry tomatoes. Cook for another 2 minutes.
- Sprinkle with pine nuts, salt, and pepper before serving.

Prep Time: 20 minutes
Servings: 1
Cooking Method: Stovetop
Nutritional Values:

- Calories: 250
- Protein: 15g
- Carbs: 20g
- Fat: 14g

Difficulty: 2/5

Ingredients:

- 1/2 cup firm tofu, cubed
- 1/2 cup broccoli florets
- 1/4 cup sliced bell peppers
- 1/4 cup snap peas
- 1 tbsp soy sauce
- 1 tbsp sesame oil
- 1 clove garlic, minced
- 1 tsp grated ginger

Procedure:

- Heat sesame oil in a pan over medium heat. Add garlic and ginger, and sauté for 1 minute.
- Add tofu and cook until golden brown, about 5 minutes.
- Add broccoli, bell peppers, and snap peas. Cook for another 5 minutes.
- Add soy sauce and toss to combine. Serve hot.

RECIPE 37: BAKED LEMON HERB SALMON

Prep Time: 20 minutes
Servings: 1
Cooking Method: Oven
Nutritional Values:

- Calories: 400
- Protein: 34g
- Carbohydrates: 2g
- Fat: 28g

Difficulty: 2/5

Ingredients:

- 1 salmon fillet (6 oz)
- 1 tbsp olive oil
- 1 tbsp lemon juice
- 1 garlic clove, minced
- 1 tsp dried dill
- 1 tsp dried parsley
- Salt and pepper to taste

Procedure:

- Preheat the oven to 375°F (190°C).
- In a small bowl, mix olive oil, lemon juice, garlic, dill, parsley, salt, and pepper.
- Place the salmon fillet on a baking sheet and brush with the herb mixture.
- Bake for 15-20 minutes or until the salmon flakes easily with a fork.

RECIPE 38: QUINOA-STUFFED BELL PEPPERS

Prep Time: 40 minutes
Servings: 1
Cooking Method: Oven
Nutritional Values:

- Calories: 350
- Protein: 15g
- Carbohydrates: 45g
- Fat: 12g

Difficulty: 3/5

Ingredients:

- 1 bell pepper
- 1/2 cup cooked quinoa
- 1/4 cup black beans, rinsed and drained
- 1/4 cup corn kernels
- 1/4 cup diced tomatoes
- 1/4 cup shredded cheddar cheese
- 1 tsp cumin
- 1 tsp chili powder
- Salt and pepper to taste

Procedure:

- Turn the oven on to 375°F, or 190°C.
- Remove the bell pepper's seeds by cutting off the top.

- Combine the cooked quinoa, diced tomatoes, black beans, corn, cumin, chili powder, and salt and pepper in a bowl.
- Place the bell pepper in a baking dish after stuffing it with the quinoa mixture.
- Top with shredded cheddar cheese.
- Bake for 25-30 minutes until the pepper is tender and the cheese is melted.

RECIPE 39: CHICKEN AND VEGETABLE STIR-FRY

Prep Time: 25 minutes
Servings: 1
Cooking Method: Stovetop
Nutritional Values:

- Calories: 350
- Protein: 25g
- Carbohydrates: 20g
- Fat: 18g

Difficulty: 2/5

Ingredients:

- 4 oz chicken breast, sliced
- 1/2 cup broccoli florets
- 1/2 cup sliced bell pepper
- 1/4 cup sliced carrots
- 1 tbsp soy sauce
- 1 tbsp sesame oil
- 1 tsp grated ginger
- 1 garlic clove, minced
- 1 tbsp sesame seeds

Procedure:

- Heat sesame oil in a large skillet over medium-high heat.
- Add garlic and ginger, and sauté for 1 minute.
- Add chicken slices and cook until no longer pink.
- Add broccoli, bell pepper, and carrots, and stir-fry for 5-7 minutes.
- Add soy sauce and stir to combine.
- Sprinkle with sesame seeds before serving.

RECIPE 40: SPINACH AND MUSHROOM STUFFED CHICKEN BREAST

Prep Time: 40 minutes
Servings: 1
Cooking Method: Oven
Nutritional Values:

- Calories: 400
- Protein: 35g
- Carbohydrates: 5g
- Fat: 25g

Difficulty: 3/5

Ingredients:

- 1 chicken breast
- 1/2 cup fresh spinach
- 1/4 cup sliced mushrooms
- 1/4 cup shredded mozzarella cheese
- 1 tbsp olive oil
- 1 tsp dried thyme
- Salt and pepper to taste

Procedure:

- Preheat the oven to 375°F (190°C).
- Butterfly the chicken breast and season with salt, pepper, and thyme.
- In a skillet, heat olive oil and sauté spinach and mushrooms until wilted.
- Stuff the chicken breast with the spinach-mushroom mixture and mozzarella cheese.
- Secure with toothpicks and place in a baking dish.
- Bake for 25-30 minutes until the chicken is cooked through.

RECIPE 41: ZUCCHINI NOODLES WITH PESTO

Prep Time: 20 minutes
Servings: 1
Cooking Method: Stovetop
Nutritional Values:

- Calories: 250
- Protein: 5g
- Carbohydrates: 15g
- Fat: 20g

Difficulty: 1/5

Ingredients:

- 2 medium zucchinis, spiralized
- 1/4 cup basil pesto
- 1 tbsp olive oil
- 1/4 cup cherry tomatoes, halved
- Salt and pepper to taste

Procedure:

- Heat olive oil in a large skillet over medium heat.
- Add zucchini noodles and cook for 3-5 minutes until tender.
- Add basil pesto and cherry tomatoes, and toss to combine.
- Season with salt and pepper.
- Serve immediately.

RECIPE 42: BALSAMIC GLAZED PORK CHOPS

Prep Time: 30 minutes
Servings: 1
Cooking Method: Stovetop
Nutritional Values:

- Calories: 400
- Protein: 30g
- Carbohydrates: 20g
- Fat: 20g

Difficulty: 2/5

Ingredients:

- 1 pork chop (6 oz)
- 1 tbsp olive oil
- 1/4 cup balsamic vinegar
- 1 tbsp honey
- 1 garlic clove, minced
- Salt and pepper to taste

Procedure:

- Heat olive oil in a skillet over medium-high heat.
- Season the pork chop with salt and pepper.
- Cook the pork chop for 4-5 minutes on each side until golden brown and cooked through.
- In a small bowl, mix balsamic vinegar, honey, and minced garlic.
- Pour the balsamic glaze over the pork chop and cook for an additional 2-3 minutes.
- Serve with your favorite side dish.

RECIPE 43: SHRIMP AND ASPARAGUS RISOTTO

Prep Time: 35 minutes
Servings: 1
Cooking Method: Stovetop
Nutritional Values:

- Calories: 500
- Protein: 25g
- Carbohydrates: 60g
- Fat: 18g

Difficulty: 3/5

Ingredients:

- 1/2 cup arborio rice
- 4 oz shrimp, peeled and deveined
- 1/2 cup asparagus, chopped
- 1/4 cup grated Parmesan cheese
- 1/2 small onion, diced
- 1 garlic clove, minced
- 2 cups low-sodium chicken broth
- 1 tbsp olive oil
- 1 tbsp butter
- Salt and pepper to taste

Procedure:

- Heat olive oil in a large skillet over medium heat. Add onion and garlic, and sauté until softened.
- Add arborio rice and cook for 1-2 minutes, stirring constantly.
- Gradually add chicken broth, one cup at a time, stirring frequently until absorbed.
- Add shrimp and asparagus during the last 5 minutes of cooking.
- Stir in butter and Parmesan cheese.
- Season with salt and pepper, and serve immediately.

RECIPE 44: STUFFED PORTOBELLO MUSHROOMS

Prep Time: 30 minutes
Servings: 1
Cooking Method: Oven
Nutritional Values:

- Calories: 250
- Protein: 10g
- Carbohydrates: 20g
- Fat: 15g

Difficulty: 2/5

Ingredients:

- 2 large portobello mushrooms
- 1/2 cup diced tomatoes
- 1/4 cup crumbled feta cheese
- 1/4 cup chopped spinach
- 1 garlic clove, minced
- 1 tbsp olive oil
- Salt and pepper to taste

Procedure:

- Preheat the oven to 375°F (190°C).
- Remove stems from the mushrooms
- and brush with olive oil.
- In a bowl, mix diced tomatoes, feta cheese, chopped spinach, minced garlic, salt, and pepper.
- Stuff the mushroom caps with the tomato mixture.
- Place on a baking sheet and bake for 20 minutes.
- Serve hot.

RECIPE 45: TURKEY AND AVOCADO WRAP

Prep Time: 10 minutes
Servings: 1
Cooking Method: No-cook
Nutritional Values:

- Calories: 350
- Protein: 25g
- Carbohydrates: 30g
- Fat: 15g

Difficulty: 1/5

Ingredients:

- 1 whole wheat tortilla
- 4 oz sliced turkey breast
- 1/2 avocado, sliced
- 1/4 cup shredded lettuce
- 1/4 cup diced tomatoes
- 1 tbsp mayonnaise
- Salt and pepper to taste

Procedure:

- Lay the tortilla flat and spread mayonnaise over it.
- Layer sliced turkey, avocado, shredded lettuce, and diced tomatoes.
- Season with salt and pepper.
- Roll up the tortilla tightly and slice in half.
- Serve immediately.

RECIPE 46: LEMON GARLIC SHRIMP PASTA

Prep Time: 20 minutes
Servings: 1
Cooking Method: Stovetop
Nutritional Values:

- Calories: 450
- Protein: 25g
- Carbohydrates: 45g
- Fat: 18g

Difficulty: 2/5

Ingredients:

- 4 oz whole wheat pasta
- 4 oz shrimp, peeled and deveined
- 1 garlic clove, minced
- 1 tbsp olive oil
- 1 tbsp lemon juice
- 1/4 cup grated Parmesan cheese
- 1 tbsp chopped parsley
- Salt and pepper to taste

Procedure:

- Cook pasta according to package instructions. Drain and set aside.
- Heat olive oil in a skillet over medium heat. Add garlic and sauté for 1 minute.
- Add shrimp and cook until pink and opaque.
- Stir in lemon juice and cooked pasta.
- Sprinkle with Parmesan cheese and chopped parsley.
- Season with salt and pepper, and serve immediately.

RECIPE 47: GRILLED LEMON HERB CHICKEN

Prep Time: 25 minutes
Servings: 1
Cooking Method: Grill
Nutritional Values:

- Calories: 300
- Protein: 30g
- Carbohydrates: 2g
- Fat: 18g

Difficulty: 2/5

Ingredients:

- 1 chicken breast
- 1 tbsp olive oil
- 1 tbsp lemon juice
- 1 tsp dried thyme
- 1 tsp dried rosemary
- 1 garlic clove, minced
- Salt and pepper to taste

Procedure:

- In a bowl, combine olive oil, lemon juice, thyme, rosemary, garlic, salt, and pepper.
- Marinate the chicken breast in the mixture for at least 15 minutes.
- Preheat the grill to medium-high heat.
- Grill the chicken for 6-7 minutes on each side or until cooked through.
- Serve with a side of grilled vegetables or salad.

RECIPE 48: BAKED COD WITH TOMATOES AND OLIVES

Prep Time: 25 minutes
Servings: 1
Cooking Method: Oven
Nutritional Values:

- Calories: 300
- Protein: 25g
- Carbohydrates: 10g
- Fat: 15g

Difficulty: 2/5

Ingredients:

- 1 cod fillet (6 oz)
- 1/4 cup cherry tomatoes, halved
- 2 tbsp sliced black olives
- 1 tbsp olive oil
- 1 garlic clove, minced
- 1 tsp dried oregano
- Salt and pepper to taste

Procedure:

- Preheat the oven to 375°F (190°C).
- Place the cod fillet in a baking dish and top with cherry tomatoes, black olives, olive oil, garlic, oregano, salt, and pepper.
- Bake for 15-20 minutes until the fish is flaky and cooked through.
- Serve with a side of steamed vegetables.

RECIPE 49: SPAGHETTI SQUASH WITH MARINARA SAUCE

Prep Time: 40 minutes
Servings: 1
Cooking Method: Oven
Nutritional Values:

- Calories: 300
- Protein: 10g
- Carbohydrates: 45g
- Fat: 10g

Difficulty: 2/5

Ingredients:

- 1 small spaghetti squash
- 1 cup marinara sauce
- 1/4 cup grated Parmesan cheese
- 1 tbsp olive oil
- 1 garlic clove, minced
- 1 tsp dried basil
- Salt and pepper to taste

Procedure:

- Preheat the oven to 375°F (190°C).
- Cut the spaghetti squash in half lengthwise and scoop out the seeds.
- Brush the inside of the squash with olive oil, and season with salt and pepper.
- Place the squash halves cut side down on a baking sheet and bake for 35-40 minutes until tender.
- Use a fork to scrape out the spaghetti-like strands.
- In a skillet, heat marinara sauce with garlic and basil.

- Toss the spaghetti squash strands with the marinara sauce and top with Parmesan cheese.
- Serve immediately.

RECIPE 50: ROASTED VEGETABLE MEDLEY

Prep Time: 35 minutes
Servings: 1
Cooking Method: Oven
Nutritional Values:

- Calories: 200
- Protein: 5g
- Carbohydrates: 30g
- Fat: 8g

Difficulty: 1/5

Ingredients:

- 1/2 cup diced sweet potato
- 1/2 cup Brussels sprouts, halved
- 1/2 cup cauliflower florets
- 1/4 cup diced red onion
- 1 tbsp olive oil
- 1 tsp dried rosemary
- Salt and pepper to taste

Procedure:

- Preheat the oven to 400°F (200°C).
- In a bowl, toss sweet potato, Brussels sprouts, cauliflower, and red onion with olive oil, rosemary, salt, and pepper.
- Spread the vegetables on a baking sheet in a single layer.
- Roast for 25-30 minutes until tender and golden brown.
- Serve as a side dish or over quinoa or rice.

FISH DELIGHTS

RECIPE 51: OMEGA-3 BLISS BAKED SALMON

Prep Time: 30 minutes
Servings: 1
Cooking Method: Baking
Nutritional Values (per serving):

- Calories: 380 kcal
- Protein: 34g
- Fat: 25g
- Carbohydrates: 2g
- Omega-3 Fatty Acids: 1.9g

Difficulty: 2/5

Ingredients:

- 1 salmon fillet (6 oz)
- 1 tbsp extra virgin olive oil
- 1 tsp minced garlic
- 1 tbsp lemon juice
- 1 tsp Dijon mustard
- 1/4 tsp dried dill
- Salt and pepper to taste

Procedure:

- Preheat oven to 375°F (190°C) and line a baking sheet with parchment paper.
- In a small bowl, mix together olive oil, garlic, lemon juice, Dijon mustard, dill, salt, and pepper.
- Place the salmon fillet on the prepared baking sheet and brush the marinade mixture over the top.
- Bake for 15-20 minutes or until the salmon flakes easily with a fork.

RECIPE 52: TURMERIC-GINGER GLAZED MAHI-MAHI

Prep Time: 25 minutes
Servings: 1
Cooking Method: Pan-Searing
Nutritional Values (per serving):

- Calories: 320 kcal
- Protein: 28g
- Fat: 15g
- Carbohydrates: 20g
- Fiber: 2g

Difficulty: 3/5

Ingredients:

- 1 mahi-mahi fillet (6 oz)
- 1 tbsp coconut oil
- 1 tsp grated ginger
- 1 tsp grated turmeric
- 1 tbsp honey
- 1 tbsp lime juice
- Salt and pepper to taste

Procedure:

- In a small bowl, mix together ginger, turmeric, honey, lime juice, salt, and pepper to form a glaze.
- Heat coconut oil in a skillet over medium-high heat.
- Season mahi-mahi fillet with salt and pepper on both sides and place it in the skillet.
- Cook for 3-4 minutes on each side until golden brown.
- Brush the glaze over the cooked mahi-mahi and cook for an additional 1-2 minutes.

RECIPE 53: LEMON-HERB GRILLED TROUT

Prep Time: 20 minutes
Servings: 1
Cooking Method: Grilling
Nutritional Values (per serving):

- Calories: 290 kcal
- Protein: 30g
- Fat: 15g
- Carbohydrates: 4g
- Fiber: 1g

Difficulty: 2/5

Ingredients:

- 1 trout fillet (6 oz)
- 1 tbsp fresh lemon juice
- 1 tsp lemon zest
- 1 tbsp chopped fresh parsley
- 1 tsp chopped fresh thyme
- 1 tsp minced garlic
- Salt and pepper to taste

Procedure:

- Preheat grill to medium heat and lightly oil the grate.
- In a small bowl, combine lemon juice, lemon zest, parsley, thyme, garlic, salt, and pepper.
- Season both sides of the trout fillet with salt and pepper, then brush with the lemon-herb mixture.
- Place the trout fillet on the grill and cook for 4-5 minutes on each side until fish flakes easily with a fork.

RECIPE 54: SAFFRON-INFUSED SEARED HALIBUT

Prep Time: 20 minutes
Servings: 1
Cooking Method: Pan-Searing
Nutritional Values (per serving):

- Calories: 310 kcal

Ingredients:

- 1 halibut fillet (6 oz)
- 1/4 tsp saffron threads
- 2 tbsp hot water
- 1 tbsp avocado oil
- 1 tsp minced shallots

- Protein: 35g
- Fat: 16g
- Carbohydrates: 2g
- Fiber: 0g
- 1/2 tsp ground coriander
- Salt and pepper to taste

Difficulty: 3/5

Procedure:

- In a small bowl, steep saffron threads in hot water for 5 minutes.
- Heat avocado oil in a skillet over medium-high heat.
- Season halibut fillet with ground coriander, salt, and pepper on both sides.
- Add minced shallots to the skillet and sauté until translucent.
- Place the halibut fillet in the skillet and sear for 3-4 minutes on each side until golden brown and cooked through.
- Pour saffron-infused water over the cooked halibut before serving.

RECIPE 55: COCONUT-CURRY POACHED COD

Prep Time: 25 minutes
Servings: 1
Cooking Method: Poaching
Nutritional Values (per serving):

- Calories: 350 kcal
- Protein: 30g
- Fat: 25g
- Carbohydrates: 8g
- Fiber: 2g

Ingredients:

- 1 cod fillet (6 oz)
- 1 cup coconut milk
- 1 tbsp red curry paste
- 1 tbsp lime juice
- 1 tsp grated ginger
- 1 tsp coconut sugar
- Salt to taste

Difficulty: 3/5

Procedure:

- In a saucepan, combine coconut milk, red curry paste, lime juice, grated ginger, coconut sugar, and salt.
- Bring the mixture to a simmer over medium heat.
- Add the cod fillet to the saucepan, ensuring it's fully submerged in the liquid.
- Poach the cod for 8-10 minutes until it flakes easily with a fork.
- Serve the cod with the poaching liquid spooned over the top.

RECIPE 56: CITRUS-MARINATED SWORDFISH SKEWERS

Prep Time: 30 minutes (plus marinating time)
Servings: 1
Cooking Method: Grilling
Nutritional Values (per serving):

- Calories: 290 kcal
- Protein: 28g
- Fat: 10g
- Carbohydrates: 18g
- Fiber: 1g

Difficulty: 3/5

Ingredients:

- 1 swordfish steak (6 oz), cut into cubes
- 1/4 cup orange juice
- 2 tbsp lime juice
- 1 tbsp honey
- 1 tsp grated orange zest
- 1 tsp grated lime zest
- 1 tsp chopped cilantro
- Salt and pepper to taste

Procedure:

- In a bowl, combine orange juice, lime juice, honey, grated orange zest, grated lime zest, chopped cilantro, salt, and pepper to make the marinade.
- Place swordfish cubes in a shallow dish and pour the marinade over them. Cover and refrigerate for at least 30 minutes.
- Preheat grill to medium-high heat.
- Thread swordfish cubes onto skewers and grill for 3-4 minutes on each side until cooked through.
- Serve hot, garnished with additional cilantro if desired.

RECIPE 57: ALMOND-CRUSTED TILAPIA WITH LEMON BUTTER SAUCE

Prep Time: 25 minutes
Servings: 1
Cooking Method: Pan-Frying
Nutritional Values (per serving):

- Calories: 330 kcal
- Protein: 32g
- Fat: 18g
- Carbohydrates: 7g
- Fiber: 2g

Difficulty: 3/5

Ingredients:

- 1 tilapia fillet (6 oz)
- 2 tbsp almond flour
- 1 tbsp grated Parmesan cheese
- 1/4 tsp paprika
- 1 egg, beaten
- 1 tbsp unsalted butter
- 1 tbsp fresh lemon juice
- 1 tsp minced garlic
- 1 tsp chopped parsley
- Salt and pepper to taste

Procedure:

- In a shallow dish, mix almond flour, grated Parmesan cheese, paprika, salt, and pepper.
- Dip tilapia fillet in beaten egg, then coat with the almond flour mixture.
- Heat butter in a skillet over medium heat. Add minced garlic and cook until fragrant.
- Add the coated tilapia fillet to the skillet and cook for 3-4 minutes on each side until golden brown and cooked through.
- Remove the tilapia from the skillet and add lemon juice, stirring to combine.
- Pour the lemon butter sauce over the tilapia and garnish with chopped parsley before serving.

RECIPE 58: CHILI-LIME GRILLED SNAPPER

Prep Time: 25 minutes
Servings: 1
Cooking Method: Grilling
Nutritional Values (per serving):

- Calories: 290 kcal
- Protein: 30g
- Fat: 15g
- Carbohydrates: 4g
- Fiber: 1g

Difficulty: 2/5

Ingredients:

- 1 snapper fillet (6 oz)
- 1 tbsp olive oil
- 1 tsp chili powder
- 1 tsp smoked paprika
- 1/2 tsp garlic powder
- 1/2 tsp onion powder
- Zest and juice of 1 lime
- Salt and pepper to taste

Procedure:

- In a small bowl, combine olive oil, chili powder, smoked paprika, garlic powder, onion powder, lime zest, lime juice, salt, and pepper to create the marinade.
- Rub the marinade over both sides of the snapper fillet and let it sit for 10-15 minutes.
- Preheat grill to medium-high heat.
- Grill the snapper fillet for 3-4 minutes on each side until grill marks appear and the fish is cooked through.
- Serve hot, garnished with additional lime wedges if desired.

RECIPE 59: PESTO-CRUSTED HADDOCK

Prep Time: 20 minutes
Servings: 1
Cooking Method: Baking
Nutritional Values (per serving):

- Calories: 320 kcal
- Protein: 30g
- Fat: 20g
- Carbohydrates: 2g
- Fiber: 1g

Difficulty: 3/5

Ingredients:

- 1 haddock fillet (6 oz)
- 2 tbsp basil pesto
- 1 tbsp grated Parmesan cheese
- 1 tbsp almond flour
- 1 tbsp olive oil
- Salt and pepper to taste

Procedure:

- Preheat oven to 375°F (190°C) and line a baking sheet with parchment paper.
- In a bowl, mix together basil pesto, grated Parmesan cheese, almond flour, salt, and pepper.
- Place the haddock fillet on the prepared baking sheet and brush with olive oil.
- Spread the pesto mixture evenly over the top of the haddock fillet.
- Bake for 12-15 minutes until the crust is golden brown and the fish is cooked through.

RECIPE 60: GARLIC-LEMON BUTTER SHRIMP SKILLET

Prep Time: 20 minutes
Servings: 1
Cooking Method: Pan-Searing
Nutritional Values (per serving):

- Calories: 110 kcal
- Protein: 15g
- Fat: 5g
- Carbohydrates: 2g
- Fiber: 0g

Difficulty: 2

Ingredients:

- 6 large shrimp, peeled and deveined
- 1 tbsp unsalted butter
- 2 cloves garlic, minced
- 1 tbsp fresh lemon juice
- 1 tsp lemon zest
- 1 tbsp chopped fresh parsley
- Salt and pepper to taste

Procedure:

- Heat butter in a skillet over medium heat.
- Add minced garlic to the skillet and cook until fragrant.
- Season shrimp with salt and pepper, then add them to the skillet.
- Cook shrimp for 2-3 minutes on each side until pink and cooked through.
- Stir in lemon juice and lemon zest, then garnish with chopped parsley before serving.

RECIPE 61: SESAME-GINGER GLAZED YELLOWTAIL

Prep Time: 25 minutes
Servings: 1
Cooking Method: Broiling
Nutritional Values (per serving):

- Calories: 280 kcal
- Protein: 30g
- Fat: 14g
- Carbohydrates: 6g
- Fiber: 1g

Difficulty: 3/5

Ingredients:

- 1 yellowtail fillet (6 oz)
- 1 tbsp sesame oil
- 1 tbsp soy sauce (low-sodium)
- 1 tsp grated ginger
- 1 tsp honey
- 1 tbsp sesame seeds
- Salt and pepper to taste

Procedure:

- Preheat the broiler and line a baking sheet with foil.
- In a bowl, whisk together sesame oil, soy sauce, grated ginger, honey, salt, and pepper.
- Place the yellowtail fillet on the prepared baking sheet.
- Brush the glaze over the fish and sprinkle with sesame seeds.
- Broil for 6-8 minutes until the fish is cooked through and caramelized.

Prep Time: 30 minutes
Servings: 1 (2 tacos)
Cooking Method: Grilling
Nutritional Values (per serving):

- Calories: 320 kcal
- Protein: 30g
- Fat: 12g
- Carbohydrates: 20g
- Fiber: 4g

Difficulty: 3

Ingredients:

- 1 red snapper fillet (6 oz)
- 2 tbsp chopped fresh cilantro
- 1 tbsp fresh lime juice
- 1 tsp lime zest
- 1/2 tsp ground cumin
- 1/2 tsp chili powder
- 1/4 tsp garlic powder
- Salt and pepper to taste

Procedure:

- Preheat grill to medium-high heat.
- In a bowl, combine chopped cilantro, lime juice, lime zest, ground cumin, chili powder, garlic powder, salt, and pepper.
- Rub the mixture over both sides of the red snapper fillet.
- Grill the red snapper fillet for 4-5 minutes on each side until it flakes easily with a fork.
- Flake the grilled fish and serve in warmed corn tortillas with your favorite toppings.

RECIPE 63: STUFFED BELL PEPPERS WITH QUINOA AND BLACK BEANS

Prep Time: 40 minutes
Servings: 1
Cooking Method: Oven
Nutritional Values:

- Calories: 350
- Protein: 15g
- Carbohydrates: 45g
- Fat: 12g

Difficulty: 3/5

Ingredients:

- 1 bell pepper
- 1/2 cup cooked quinoa
- 1/4 cup black beans, rinsed and drained
- 1/4 cup corn kernels
- 1/4 cup diced tomatoes
- 1/4 cup shredded cheddar cheese
- 1 tsp cumin
- 1 tsp chili powder
- Salt and pepper to taste

Procedure:

- Preheat the oven to 375°F (190°C).
- Cut the top off the bell pepper and remove the seeds.
- In a bowl, mix cooked quinoa, black beans, corn, diced tomatoes, cumin, chili powder, salt, and pepper.
- Stuff the bell pepper with the quinoa mixture and place in a baking dish.
- Top with shredded cheddar cheese.
- Bake for 25-30 minutes until the pepper is tender and the cheese is melted.

RECIPE 64: SPINACH AND RICOTTA STUFFED PORTOBELLO MUSHROOMS

Prep Time: 30 minutes
Servings: 1
Cooking Method: Oven
Nutritional Values:

- Calories: 300
- Protein: 15g
- Carbohydrates: 10g
- Fat: 20g

Difficulty: 2/5

Ingredients:

- 2 large portobello mushrooms
- 1/2 cup fresh spinach, chopped
- 1/4 cup ricotta cheese
- 1 garlic clove, minced
- 1 tbsp olive oil
- Salt and pepper to taste
- 1/4 cup grated Parmesan cheese

Procedure:

- Preheat the oven to 375°F (190°C).
- Remove the stems from the mushrooms and brush with olive oil.
- In a bowl, mix chopped spinach, ricotta cheese, minced garlic, salt, and pepper.
- Stuff the mushroom caps with the spinach-ricotta mixture and top with grated Parmesan cheese.
- Place on a baking sheet and bake for 20 minutes.

RECIPE 65: EGGPLANT PARMESAN

Prep Time: 45 minutes
Servings: 1
Cooking Method: Oven
Nutritional Values:

- Calories: 400
- Protein: 20g
- Carbohydrates: 35g
- Fat: 20g

Difficulty: 3/5

Ingredients:

- 1 small eggplant, sliced into rounds
- 1/2 cup marinara sauce
- 1/4 cup shredded mozzarella cheese
- 1/4 cup grated Parmesan cheese
- 1/4 cup breadcrumbs
- 1 egg, beaten
- 1 tbsp olive oil
- Salt and pepper to taste

Procedure:

- Preheat the oven to 375°F (190°C).
- Dip eggplant slices in beaten egg, then coat with breadcrumbs.
- Heat olive oil in a skillet over medium heat and fry the eggplant slices until golden brown.
- Layer fried eggplant, marinara sauce, mozzarella, and Parmesan cheese in a baking dish.
- Repeat layers and bake for 20-25 minutes until the cheese is melted and bubbly.

RECIPE 66: CHICKPEA AND SPINACH CURRY

Prep Time: 30 minutes
Servings: 1
Cooking Method: Stovetop
Nutritional Values:

- Calories: 350
- Protein: 12g
- Carbohydrates: 35g

Ingredients:

- 1/2 cup canned chickpeas, rinsed and drained
- 1 cup fresh spinach
- 1/2 cup diced tomatoes
- 1/4 cup coconut milk
- 1 tbsp olive oil
- 1 garlic clove, minced

- Fat: 18g

Difficulty: 2/5

- 1 tsp curry powder
- 1/2 tsp ground cumin
- Salt and pepper to taste

Procedure:

- Heat olive oil in a skillet over medium heat. Add garlic and sauté for 1 minute.
- Add chickpeas, diced tomatoes, curry powder, and cumin, and cook for 5 minutes.
- Stir in spinach and coconut milk, and cook until the spinach is wilted.
- Season with salt and pepper.
- Serve with a side of rice or naan bread.

RECIPE 67: LENTIL AND VEGETABLE STEW

Prep Time: 40 minutes
Servings: 1
Cooking Method: Stovetop
Nutritional Values:

- Calories: 300
- Protein: 15g
- Carbohydrates: 45g
- Fat: 8g

Difficulty: 2/5

Ingredients:

- 1/2 cup lentils, rinsed
- 1/2 cup diced carrots
- 1/2 cup diced celery
- 1/2 cup diced tomatoes
- 1/4 cup diced onion
- 2 cups vegetable broth
- 1 garlic clove, minced
- 1 tbsp olive oil
- 1 tsp dried thyme
- Salt and pepper to taste

Procedure:

- Heat olive oil in a pot over medium heat. Add garlic and onion, and sauté until softened.
- Add carrots, celery, and tomatoes, and cook for 5 minutes.
- Add lentils, vegetable broth, thyme, salt, and pepper.
- Bring to a boil, then reduce heat and simmer for 30 minutes until lentils are tender.
- Serve hot.

RECIPE 68: GRILLED VEGETABLE SKEWERS

Prep Time: 30 minutes
Servings: 1
Cooking Method: Grill
Nutritional Values:

- Calories: 200
- Protein: 4g
- Carbohydrates: 20g
- Fat: 12g

Difficulty: 2/5

Ingredients:

- 1/2 zucchini, sliced
- 1/2 bell pepper, cut into chunks
- 1/2 red onion, cut into chunks
- 4 cherry tomatoes
- 1 tbsp olive oil
- 1 tsp dried oregano
- Salt and pepper to taste

Procedure:

- Preheat the grill to medium-high heat.
- Thread zucchini, bell pepper, red onion, and cherry tomatoes onto skewers.
- Brush with olive oil and season with oregano, salt, and pepper.
- Grill for 10-15 minutes, turning occasionally, until vegetables are tender and slightly charred.
- Serve with a side of quinoa or couscous.

RECIPE 69: VEGAN STUFFED ACORN SQUASH

Prep Time: 45 minutes
Servings: 1
Cooking Method: Oven
Nutritional Values:

- Calories: 350
- Protein: 6g
- Carbohydrates: 60g
- Fat: 12g

Difficulty: 3/5

Ingredients:

- 1 small acorn squash
- 1/2 cup cooked wild rice
- 1/4 cup chopped walnuts
- 1/4 cup dried cranberries
- 1 tbsp olive oil
- 1 tsp dried sage
- Salt and pepper to taste

Procedure:

- Preheat the oven to 375°F (190°C).
- Cut the acorn squash in half and remove the seeds.
- Brush with olive oil and season with salt and pepper.
- Place cut side down on a baking sheet and bake for 30 minutes.
- In a bowl, mix cooked wild rice, chopped walnuts, dried cranberries, sage, salt, and pepper.
- Stuff the squash halves with the rice mixture and bake for an additional 15 minutes.

- Serve hot.

RECIPE 70: CAULIFLOWER TACOS WITH AVOCADO CREMA

Prep Time: 30 minutes
Servings: 1
Cooking Method: Oven
Nutritional Values:

- Calories: 300
- Protein: 8g
- Carbohydrates: 35g
- Fat: 15g

Difficulty: 2/5

Ingredients:

- 1/2 head of cauliflower, cut into florets
- 1 tbsp olive oil
- 1 tsp smoked paprika
- 1 tsp cumin
- Salt and pepper to taste
- 1 small avocado
- 1 tbsp lime juice
- 1/4 cup plain Greek yogurt
- 2 small corn tortillas
- 1/4 cup shredded red cabbage
- Fresh cilantro for garnish

Procedure:

- Preheat the oven to 400°F (200°C).
- Toss cauliflower florets with olive oil, smoked paprika, cumin, salt, and pepper.
- Spread on a baking sheet and roast for 20 minutes until tender.
- In a blender, combine avocado, lime juice, Greek yogurt, salt, and pepper until smooth.
- Warm the corn tortillas and fill with roasted cauliflower, shredded red cabbage, and avocado crema.
- Garnish with fresh cilantro and serve.

RECIPE 71: MUSHROOM AND BARLEY RISOTTO

Prep Time: 40 minutes
Servings: 1
Cooking Method: Stovetop
Nutritional Values:

- Calories: 350
- Protein: 10g
- Carbohydrates: 55g
- Fat: 10g

Difficulty: 3/5

Ingredients:

- 1/2 cup pearl barley
- 1 cup vegetable broth
- 1/2 cup sliced mushrooms
- 1/4 cup diced onion
- 1 garlic clove, minced
- 1 tbsp olive oil
- 1 tbsp nutritional yeast
- 1 tsp dried thyme
- Salt and pepper to taste

Procedure:

- Heat olive oil in a pot over medium heat. Add garlic and onion, and sauté until softened.
- Add sliced mushrooms and cook until browned.
- Stir in pearl barley, vegetable broth, thyme, salt, and pepper.
- Bring to a boil, then reduce heat and simmer for 30 minutes until barley is tender.
- Stir in nutritional yeast and serve hot.

RECIPE 72: SWEET POTATO AND BLACK BEAN ENCHILADAS

Prep Time: 40 minutes
Servings: 1
Cooking Method: Oven
Nutritional Values:

- Calories: 400
- Protein: 15g
- Carbohydrates: 60g
- Fat: 12g

Difficulty: 3/5

Ingredients:

- 1 small sweet potato, diced
- 1/2 cup black beans, rinsed and drained
- 1/4 cup corn kernels
- 1/2 cup enchilada sauce
- 1/4 cup shredded cheddar cheese
- 2 small whole wheat tortillas
- 1 tbsp olive oil
- 1 tsp cumin
- Salt and pepper to taste

Procedure:

- Preheat the oven to 375°F (190°C).
- Toss diced sweet potato with olive oil, cumin, salt, and pepper, and roast for 20 minutes until tender.
- In a bowl, mix roasted sweet potato, black beans, corn, and half of the enchilada sauce.
- Fill the tortillas with the sweet potato mixture, roll up, and place in a baking dish.
- Pour remaining enchilada sauce over the top and sprinkle with shredded cheddar cheese.
- Bake for 15 minutes until the cheese is melted and bubbly.

RECIPE 73: ANTI-INFLAMMATORY TURMERIC CHICKEN SOUP

Prep Time: 30 minutes
Servings: 4
Cooking Method: Stovetop
Nutritional Values:

- Calories: 200
- Protein: 20g
- Carbohydrates: 15g
- Fat: 8g

Difficulty: 2/5

Ingredients:

- 1 boneless, skinless chicken breast
- 1 tbsp olive oil
- 1 small onion, diced
- 2 garlic cloves, minced
- 1 tsp ground turmeric
- 1 tsp ground ginger
- 2 carrots, sliced
- 2 celery stalks, sliced
- 1 cup baby spinach
- 4 cups low-sodium chicken broth
- Salt and pepper to taste

Procedure:

- Heat olive oil in a large pot over medium heat. Add the diced onion and minced garlic, sauté until softened.
- Add the ground turmeric and ground ginger, stirring to combine.
- Add the chicken breast and cook until lightly browned on both sides, about 5 minutes.
- Pour in the chicken broth and bring to a boil. Reduce the heat to low and simmer for 20 minutes, until the chicken is cooked through.
- Remove the chicken breast, shred it with two forks, and return it to the pot.
- Add the sliced carrots, celery, and baby spinach. Cook for an additional 10 minutes, until the vegetables are tender.
- Season with salt and pepper to taste.

RECIPE 74: CURRIED LENTIL AND SWEET POTATO STEW

Prep Time: 40 minutes
Servings: 4
Cooking Method: Stovetop
Nutritional Values:

- Calories: 300
- Protein: 12g
- Carbohydrates: 45g
- Fat: 10g

Difficulty: 2/5

Ingredients:

- 1 cup red lentils, rinsed
- 1 large sweet potato, diced
- 1 small onion, diced
- 2 garlic cloves, minced
- 1 tbsp olive oil
- 1 tbsp curry powder
- 1 tsp ground cumin
- 1 can (14.5 oz) diced tomatoes

- 4 cups vegetable broth
- 1 cup coconut milk
- 1 cup chopped kale
- Salt and pepper to taste

Procedure:

- Heat olive oil in a large pot over medium heat. Add the onion and garlic, sauté until softened.
- Add the curry powder and ground cumin, stirring to combine.
- Add the diced sweet potato and red lentils, stirring to coat with the spices.
- Pour in the vegetable broth and diced tomatoes. Bring to a boil, then reduce the heat and simmer for 25 minutes, until the lentils and sweet potato are tender.
- Stir in the coconut milk and chopped kale. Cook for an additional 5 minutes, until the kale is wilted.
- Season with salt and pepper to taste.

RECIPE 75: GINGER CARROT SOUP

Prep Time: 30 minutes
Servings: 4
Cooking Method: Stovetop
Nutritional Values:

- Calories: 250
- Protein: 3g
- Carbohydrates: 30g
- Fat: 14g

Difficulty: 2/5

Ingredients:

- 1 tbsp olive oil
- 1 small onion, chopped
- 2 lbs carrots, peeled and chopped
- 1 tbsp fresh ginger, grated
- 4 cups vegetable broth
- 1 cup coconut milk
- Salt and pepper to taste
- Fresh cilantro for garnish

Procedure:

- Heat olive oil in a large pot over medium heat. Add the chopped onion and sauté until softened.
- Add the chopped carrots and grated ginger, stirring to combine.
- Pour in the vegetable broth and bring to a boil. Reduce the heat and simmer for 20 minutes, until the carrots are tender.
- Using an immersion blender, puree the soup until smooth.
- Stir in the coconut milk and season with salt and pepper.
- Serve garnished with fresh cilantro.

RECIPE 76: BUTTERNUT SQUASH AND APPLE SOUP

Prep Time: 35 minutes
Servings: 4
Cooking Method: Stovetop
Nutritional Values:

- Calories: 220
- Protein: 2g
- Carbohydrates: 35g
- Fat: 9g

Difficulty: 2/5

Ingredients:

- 1 tbsp olive oil
- 1 small onion, diced
- 1 butternut squash, peeled and cubed
- 2 apples, peeled and chopped
- 4 cups vegetable broth
- 1/2 cup coconut milk
- 1 tsp ground cinnamon
- Salt and pepper to taste
- Pumpkin seeds for garnish

Procedure:

- Heat olive oil in a large pot over medium heat. Add the diced onion and sauté until softened.
- Add the butternut squash and apples, stirring to combine.
- Pour in the vegetable broth and bring to a boil. Reduce the heat and simmer for 20 minutes, until the squash and apples are tender.
- Using an immersion blender, puree the soup until smooth.
- Stir in the coconut milk and ground cinnamon. Season with salt and pepper.
- Serve garnished with pumpkin seeds.

RECIPE 77: MOROCCAN CHICKPEA STEW

Prep Time: 45 minutes
Servings: 4
Cooking Method: Stovetop
Nutritional Values:

- Calories: 280
- Protein: 8g
- Carbohydrates: 45g
- Fat: 9g

Difficulty: 3/5

Ingredients:

- 1 tbsp olive oil
- 1 small onion, diced
- 2 garlic cloves, minced
- 1 tsp ground cumin
- 1 tsp ground coriander
- 1/2 tsp ground cinnamon
- 1 can (14.5 oz) chickpeas, rinsed and drained
- 1 can (14.5 oz) diced tomatoes
- 1 cup diced butternut squash
- 4 cups vegetable broth
- 1/4 cup chopped fresh cilantro
- Salt and pepper to taste

Procedure:

- Heat olive oil in a large pot over medium heat. Add the onion and garlic, sauté until softened.
- Add the ground cumin, coriander, and cinnamon, stirring to combine.
- Add the chickpeas, diced tomatoes, butternut squash, and vegetable broth. Bring to a boil, then reduce the heat and simmer for 30 minutes, until the squash is tender.
- Stir in the chopped cilantro and season with salt and pepper.
- Serve hot.

RECIPE 78: RED LENTIL AND COCONUT SOUP

Prep Time: 30 minutes
Servings: 4
Cooking Method: Stovetop
Nutritional Values:

- Calories: 350
- Protein: 12g
- Carbohydrates: 40g
- Fat: 18g

Difficulty: 2/5

Ingredients:

- 1 tbsp olive oil
- 1 small onion, chopped
- 2 garlic cloves, minced
- 1 cup red lentils, rinsed
- 4 cups vegetable broth
- 1 can (14 oz) coconut milk
- 1 tbsp curry powder
- 1 tsp ground turmeric
- Salt and pepper to taste
- Fresh cilantro for garnish

Procedure:

- Heat olive oil in a large pot over medium heat. Add the chopped onion and minced garlic, sauté until softened.
- Add the curry powder and ground turmeric, stirring to combine.
- Add the red lentils and vegetable broth. Bring to a boil, then reduce the heat and simmer for 20 minutes, until the lentils are tender.
- Stir in the coconut milk and season with salt and pepper.
- Serve garnished with fresh cilantro.

RECIPE 79: ITALIAN MINESTRONE SOUP

Prep Time: 45 minutes
Servings: 4
Cooking Method: Stovetop
Nutritional Values:

- Calories: 300
- Protein: 10g

Ingredients:

- 1 tbsp olive oil
- 1 small onion, diced
- 2 garlic cloves, minced
- 2 carrots, diced
- 2 celery stalks, diced

- Carbohydrates: 45g
- Fat: 8g

Difficulty: 2/5

- 1 zucchini, diced
- 1 can (14.5 oz) diced tomatoes
- 4 cups vegetable broth
- 1 can (14.5 oz) kidney beans, rinsed and drained
- 1/2 cup pasta (optional)
- 1 tsp dried basil
- 1 tsp dried oregano
- Salt and pepper to taste
- Fresh parsley for garnish

Procedure:

- Heat olive oil in a large pot over medium heat. Add the onion and garlic, sauté until softened.
- Add the carrots, celery, and zucchini, stirring to combine.
- Pour in the diced tomatoes and vegetable broth. Bring to a boil, then reduce the heat and simmer for 20 minutes.
- Add the kidney beans, pasta (if using), dried basil, and dried oregano. Simmer for an additional 10 minutes, until the pasta is tender.
- Season with salt and pepper.
- Serve garnished with fresh parsley.

RECIPE 80: HEARTY VEGETABLE STEW

Prep Time: 50 minutes
Servings: 4
Cooking Method: Stovetop
Nutritional Values:

- Calories: 280
- Protein: 6g
- Carbohydrates: 50g
- Fat: 7g

Difficulty: 3/5

Ingredients:

- 1 tbsp olive oil
- 1 small onion, diced
- 2 garlic cloves, minced
- 2 carrots, sliced
- 2 celery stalks, sliced
- 1 sweet potato, diced
- 1 zucchini, diced
- 1 cup green beans, trimmed and cut into pieces
- 4 cups vegetable broth
- 1 can (14.5 oz) diced tomatoes
- 1 tsp dried thyme
- 1 tsp dried rosemary
- Salt and pepper to taste

Procedure:

- Heat olive oil in a large pot over medium heat. Add the onion and garlic, sauté until softened.
- Add the carrots, celery, sweet potato, zucchini, and green beans, stirring to combine.
- Pour in the vegetable broth and diced tomatoes. Bring to a boil, then reduce the heat and simmer for 30 minutes, until the vegetables are tender.
- Stir in the dried thyme and rosemary. Season with salt and pepper.
- Serve hot.

BREAD

RECIPE 81: ALMOND FLOUR BANANA BREAD

Prep Time: 15 minutes
Servings: 1 loaf (about 8 slices)
Cooking Method: Baking
Nutritional Values (per slice):

- Calories: 150 kcal
- Protein: 5g
- Fat: 9g
- Carbohydrates: 15g
- Fiber: 3g

Difficulty: 2/5

Ingredients:

- 1 cup almond flour
- 2 ripe bananas, mashed
- 2 eggs
- 1/4 cup honey or maple syrup
- 1 teaspoon vanilla extract
- 1/2 teaspoon baking soda
- 1/2 teaspoon cinnamon
- Pinch of salt

Procedure:

- Preheat oven to 350°F (175°C). Grease a loaf pan with coconut oil or line it with parchment paper.
- In a mixing bowl, combine almond flour, mashed bananas, eggs, honey or maple syrup, vanilla extract, baking soda, cinnamon, and salt. ix until well combined and pour the batter into the prepared loaf pan.
- Bake for 40-45 minutes, or until a toothpick inserted into the center comes out clean.
- Allow the banana bread to cool in the pan for 10 minutes, then transfer it to a wire rack to cool completely before slicing.

RECIPE 82: QUINOA FLOUR ZUCCHINI BREAD

Prep Time: 20 minutes
Servings: 1 loaf (about 8 slices)
Cooking Method: Baking
Nutritional Values (per slice):

- Calories: 130 kcal
- Protein: 3g
- Fat: 6g
- Carbohydrates: 18g
- Fiber: 2g

Difficulty: 3/5

Ingredients:

- 1 cup quinoa flour
- 1 teaspoon baking powder
- 1/2 teaspoon baking soda
- 1/4 teaspoon salt
- 1 teaspoon cinnamon
- 2 eggs
- 1/4 cup honey or maple syrup
- 1/4 cup coconut oil, melted
- 1 teaspoon vanilla extract
- 1 cup grated zucchini

Procedure:

- Preheat oven to 350°F (175°C). Grease a loaf pan with coconut oil or line it with parchment paper.
- In a large bowl, whisk together quinoa flour, baking powder, baking soda, salt, and cinnamon.
- In another bowl, beat eggs and mix in honey or maple syrup, melted coconut oil, and vanilla extract.
- Stir the wet ingredients into the dry ingredients until well combined. Fold in the grated zucchini.
- Pour the batter into the prepared loaf pan.
- Bake for 40-45 minutes, or until a toothpick inserted into the center comes out clean.
- Allow the zucchini bread to cool in the pan for 10 minutes, then transfer it to a wire rack to cool completely before slicing.

RECIPE 83: OAT FLOUR BLUEBERRY BREAD

Prep Time: 15 minutes
Servings: 1 loaf (about 8 slices)
Cooking Method: Baking
Nutritional Values (per slice):

- Calories: 150 kcal
- Protein: 4g
- Fat: 3g
- Carbohydrates: 28g
- Fiber: 3g

Difficulty: 2/5

Ingredients:

- 1 1/2 cups oat flour
- 1/2 teaspoon baking soda
- 1/2 teaspoon baking powder
- Pinch of salt
- 2 ripe bananas, mashed
- 1/4 cup honey or maple syrup
- 1/4 cup unsweetened applesauce
- 2 eggs
- 1 teaspoon vanilla extract
- 1 cup fresh or frozen blueberries

Procedure:

- Preheat oven to 350°F (175°C). Grease a loaf pan with coconut oil or line it with parchment paper.
- In a large bowl, whisk together oat flour, baking soda, baking powder, and salt.
- In another bowl, mix together mashed bananas, honey or maple syrup, unsweetened applesauce, eggs, and vanilla extract until well combined.
- Add the wet ingredients to the dry ingredients and stir until just combined.
- Gently fold in the blueberries.
- Pour the batter into the prepared loaf pan.
- Bake for 45-50 minutes, or until a toothpick inserted into the center comes out clean.
- Allow the blueberry bread to cool in the pan for 10 minutes, then transfer it to a wire rack to cool completely before slicing.

RECIPE 84: BUCKWHEAT FLOUR PUMPKIN BREAD

Prep Time: 20 minutes
Servings: 1 loaf (about 8 slices)
Cooking Method: Baking
Nutritional Values (per slice):

- Calories: 170 kcal
- Protein: 4g
- Fat: 6g
- Carbohydrates: 26g
- Fiber: 3g

Difficulty: 3/5

Ingredients:

- 1 1/2 cups buckwheat flour
- 1 teaspoon baking soda
- 1/2 teaspoon baking powder
- 1/2 teaspoon ground cinnamon
- 1/4 teaspoon ground nutmeg
- Pinch of salt
- 1 cup pumpkin puree
- 1/3 cup honey or maple syrup
- 1/4 cup coconut oil, melted
- 2 eggs
- 1 teaspoon vanilla extract

Procedure:

- Preheat oven to 350°F (175°C). Grease a loaf pan with coconut oil or line it with parchment paper.
- In a large bowl, whisk together buckwheat flour, baking soda, baking powder, cinnamon, nutmeg, and salt.
- In another bowl, mix together pumpkin puree, honey or maple syrup, melted coconut oil, eggs, and vanilla extract until well combined.
- Add the wet ingredients to the dry ingredients and stir until just combined.
- Pour the batter into the prepared loaf pan.
- Bake for 45-50 minutes, or until a toothpick inserted into the center comes out clean.
- Allow the pumpkin bread to cool in the pan for 10 minutes, then transfer it to a wire rack to cool completely before slicing.

RECIPE 85: SPELT FLOUR DATE NUT BREAD

Prep Time: 20 minutes
Servings: 1 loaf (about 8 slices)
Cooking Method: Baking
Nutritional Values (per slice):

- Calories: 180 kcal
- Protein: 4g
- Fat: 8g
- Carbohydrates: 24g
- Fiber: 3g

Difficulty: 3/5

Ingredients:

- 1 1/2 cups spelt flour
- 1 teaspoon baking powder
- 1/2 teaspoon baking soda
- Pinch of salt
- 1/4 cup coconut oil, melted
- 1/4 cup honey or maple syrup
- 2 eggs
- 1 teaspoon vanilla extract
- 1/2 cup chopped dates

- 1/2 cup chopped nuts (such as walnuts or pecans)

Procedure:

- Preheat oven to 350°F (175°C). Grease a loaf pan with coconut oil or line it with parchment paper.
- In a large bowl, whisk together spelt flour, baking powder, baking soda, and salt.
- In another bowl, mix together melted coconut oil, honey or maple syrup, eggs, and vanilla extract until well combined.
- Add the wet ingredients to the dry ingredients and stir until just combined.
- Fold in chopped dates and nuts.
- Pour the batter into the prepared loaf pan.
- Bake for 45-50 minutes, or until a toothpick inserted into the center comes out clean.
- Allow the date nut bread to cool in the pan for 10 minutes, then transfer it to a wire rack to cool completely before slicing.

RECIPE 86: TEFF FLOUR CINNAMON RAISIN BREAD

Prep Time: 20 minutes
Servings: 1 loaf (about 8 slices)
Cooking Method: Baking
Nutritional Values (per slice):

- Calories: 170 kcal
- Protein: 4g
- Fat: 7g
- Carbohydrates: 25g
- Fiber: 3g

Difficulty: 3/5

Ingredients:

- 1 1/2 cups teff flour
- 1 teaspoon baking powder
- 1/2 teaspoon baking soda
- 1/2 teaspoon ground cinnamon
- Pinch of salt
- 1/4 cup coconut oil, melted
- 1/4 cup honey or maple syrup
- 2 eggs
- 1 teaspoon vanilla extract
- 1/2 cup raisins

Procedure:

- Preheat oven to 350°F (175°C). Grease a loaf pan with coconut oil or line it with parchment paper.
- In a large bowl, whisk together teff flour, baking powder, baking soda, cinnamon, and salt.
- In another bowl, mix together melted coconut oil, honey or maple syrup, eggs, and vanilla extract until well combined.
- Add the wet ingredients to the dry ingredients and stir until just combined.
- Fold in raisins.
- Pour the batter into the prepared loaf pan.

- Bake for 45-50 minutes, or until a toothpick inserted into the center comes out clean.
- Allow the cinnamon raisin bread to cool in the pan for 10 minutes, then transfer it to a wire rack to cool completely before slicing.

RECIPE 87: MILLET FLOUR CRANBERRY ORANGE BREAD

Prep Time: 20 minutes
Servings: 1 loaf (about 8 slices)
Cooking Method: Baking
Nutritional Values (per slice):

- Calories: 180 kcal
- Protein: 4g
- Fat: 8g
- Carbohydrates: 25g
- Fiber: 3g

Difficulty: 3/5

Ingredients:

- 1 1/2 cups millet flour
- 1 teaspoon baking powder
- 1/2 teaspoon baking soda
- Pinch of salt
- 1/4 cup coconut oil, melted
- 1/4 cup honey or maple syrup
- 2 eggs
- 1 teaspoon vanilla extract
- Zest of 1 orange
- 1/2 cup fresh cranberries, chopped

Procedure:

- Preheat oven to 350°F (175°C). Grease a loaf pan with coconut oil or line it with parchment paper.
- In a large bowl, whisk together millet flour, baking powder, baking soda, and salt.
- In another bowl, mix together melted coconut oil, honey or maple syrup, eggs, vanilla extract, and orange zest until well combined.
- Add the wet ingredients to the dry ingredients and stir until just combined.
- Fold in chopped cranberries.
- Pour the batter into the prepared loaf pan.
- Bake for 45-50 minutes, or until a toothpick inserted into the center comes out clean.
- Allow the cranberry orange bread to cool in the pan for 10 minutes, then transfer it to a wire rack to cool completely before slicing.

RECIPE 88: BUCKWHEAT BANANA BREAD WITH WALNUTS

Prep Time: 20 minutes
Servings: 1 loaf (about 8 slices)
Cooking Method: Baking
Nutritional Values (per slice):

- Calories: 190 kcal

Ingredients:

- 1 1/2 cups buckwheat flour
- 1 teaspoon baking powder
- 1/2 teaspoon baking soda
- Pinch of salt

- Protein: 5g
- Fat: 9g
- Carbohydrates: 25g
- Fiber: 3g

Difficulty: 3/5

- 1/4 cup coconut oil, melted
- 1/4 cup honey or maple syrup
- 2 ripe bananas, mashed
- 2 eggs
- 1 teaspoon vanilla extract
- 1/2 cup chopped walnuts

Procedure:

- Preheat oven to 350°F (175°C). Grease a loaf pan with coconut oil or line it with parchment paper.
- In a large bowl, whisk together buckwheat flour, baking powder, baking soda, and salt.
- In another bowl, mix together melted coconut oil, honey or maple syrup, mashed bananas, eggs, and vanilla extract until well combined.
- Add the wet ingredients to the dry ingredients and stir until just combined.
- Fold in chopped walnuts.
- Pour the batter into the prepared loaf pan.
- Bake for 45-50 minutes, or until a toothpick inserted into the center comes out clean.
- Allow the banana walnut bread to cool in the pan for 10 minutes, then transfer it to a wire rack to cool completely before slicing.

RECIPE 89: SORGHUM FLOUR ROSEMARY OLIVE BREAD

Prep Time: 20 minutes
Servings: 1 loaf (about 8 slices)
Cooking Method: Baking
Nutritional Values (per slice):

- Calories: 180 kcal
- Protein: 5g
- Fat: 9g
- Carbohydrates: 20g
- Fiber: 3g

Difficulty: 3/5

Ingredients:

- 1 1/2 cups sorghum flour
- 1 teaspoon baking powder
- 1/2 teaspoon baking soda
- Pinch of salt
- 1/4 cup olive oil
- 1/4 cup unsweetened almond milk
- 2 eggs
- 1 teaspoon honey
- 1 tablespoon chopped fresh rosemary
- 1/2 cup chopped olives (black or green)

Procedure:

- Preheat oven to 350°F (175°C). Grease a loaf pan with olive oil or line it with parchment paper.
- In a large bowl, whisk together sorghum flour, baking powder, baking soda, and salt.

- In another bowl, mix together olive oil, almond milk, eggs, and honey until well combined.
- Add the wet ingredients to the dry ingredients and stir until just combined.
- Fold in chopped fresh rosemary and olives.
- Pour the batter into the prepared loaf pan.
- Bake for 45-50 minutes, or until a toothpick inserted into the center comes out clean.
- Allow the rosemary olive bread to cool in the pan for 10 minutes, then transfer it to a wire rack to cool completely before slicing.

RECIPE 90: AMARANTH FLOUR SUNFLOWER SEED BREAD

Prep Time: 20 minutes
Servings: 1 loaf (about 8 slices)
Cooking Method: Baking
Nutritional Values (per slice):

- Calories: 190 kcal
- Protein: 5g
- Fat: 9g
- Carbohydrates: 21g
- Fiber: 3g

Difficulty: 3/5

Ingredients:

- 1 1/2 cups amaranth flour
- 1 teaspoon baking powder
- 1/2 teaspoon baking soda
- Pinch of salt
- 1/4 cup coconut oil, melted
- 1/4 cup unsweetened almond milk
- 2 eggs
- 1 teaspoon honey or maple syrup
- 1/4 cup raw sunflower seeds

Procedure:

- Preheat oven to 350°F (175°C). Grease a loaf pan with coconut oil or line it with parchment paper.
- In a large bowl, whisk together amaranth flour, baking powder, baking soda, and salt.
- In another bowl, mix together melted coconut oil, almond milk, eggs, and honey until well combined.
- Add the wet ingredients to the dry ingredients and stir until just combined.
- Fold in raw sunflower seeds.
- Pour the batter into the prepared loaf pan.
- Bake for 45-50 minutes, or until a toothpick inserted into the center comes out clean.
- Allow the sunflower seed bread to cool in the pan for 10 minutes, then transfer it to a wire rack to cool completely before slicing.

SNACKS

RECIPE 91: ALMOND ENERGY BITES

Prep Time: 15 minutes
Servings: 12 bites
Cooking Method: No cooking required
Nutritional Values:

- Calories: 120 per bite
- Protein: 3g
- Carbohydrates: 10g
- Fat: 8g

Difficulty: 1/5

Ingredients:

- 1 cup almond flour
- 1/2 cup almond butter
- 1/4 cup honey
- 1/2 cup shredded coconut
- 1/4 cup dark chocolate chips
- 1 tsp vanilla extract

Procedure:

- In a large bowl, combine almond flour, almond butter, honey, shredded coconut, dark chocolate chips, and vanilla extract.
- Mix well until all ingredients are fully combined.
- Roll the mixture into 1-inch balls.
- Refrigerate for at least 30 minutes before serving.

RECIPE 92: AVOCADO HUMMUS

Prep Time: 10 minutes
Servings: 4
Cooking Method: No cooking required
Nutritional Values:

- Calories: 180 per serving
- Protein: 4g
- Carbohydrates: 16g
- Fat: 12g

Difficulty: 1/5

Ingredients:

- 1 ripe avocado
- 1 can (15 oz) chickpeas, drained and rinsed
- 2 tbsp tahini
- 2 tbsp olive oil
- 1 garlic clove, minced
- 1 lemon, juiced
- Salt and pepper to taste

Procedure:

- In a food processor, combine avocado, chickpeas, tahini, olive oil, minced garlic, and lemon juice.
- Blend until smooth.
- Season with salt and pepper to taste.

- Serve with veggie sticks or whole grain crackers.

RECIPE 93: BAKED KALE CHIPS

Prep Time: 5 minutes
Servings: 4
Cooking Method: Oven
Nutritional Values:

- Calories: 50 per serving
- Protein: 2g
- Carbohydrates: 7g
- Fat: 2g

Difficulty: 1/5

Ingredients:

- 1 bunch kale, washed and dried
- 1 tbsp olive oil
- 1/2 tsp sea salt

Procedure:

- Preheat oven to 350°F (175°C).
- Remove kale leaves from stems and tear into bite-sized pieces.
- Toss kale with olive oil and sea salt.
- Spread evenly on a baking sheet.
- Bake for 10-15 minutes, until edges are browned but not burnt.

RECIPE 94: CHIA SEED PUDDING

Prep Time: 5 minutes (plus overnight chilling)
Servings: 2
Cooking Method: No cooking required
Nutritional Values:

- Calories: 180 per serving
- Protein: 4g
- Carbohydrates: 18g
- Fat: 9g

Difficulty: 1/5

Ingredients:

- 1/4 cup chia seeds
- 1 cup almond milk
- 1 tbsp honey
- 1/2 tsp vanilla extract

Procedure:

- In a bowl, mix chia seeds, almond milk, honey, and vanilla extract.
- Stir well to combine.
- Refrigerate overnight or for at least 4 hours.
- Serve chilled.

RECIPE 95: QUINOA SALAD CUPS

Prep Time: 20 minutes
Servings: 4
Cooking Method: No cooking required
Nutritional Values:

- Calories: 220 per serving
- Protein: 6g
- Carbohydrates: 20g
- Fat: 12g

Difficulty: 2/5

Ingredients:

- 1 cup cooked quinoa
- 1/2 cup cherry tomatoes, halved
- 1/4 cup cucumber, diced
- 1/4 cup red onion, diced
- 1/4 cup feta cheese, crumbled
- 2 tbsp olive oil
- 1 tbsp lemon juice
- Salt and pepper to taste

Procedure:

- In a bowl, combine cooked quinoa, cherry tomatoes, cucumber, red onion, and feta cheese.
- Drizzle with olive oil and lemon juice.
- Season with salt and pepper to taste.
- Spoon into small cups or bowls for serving.

RECIPE 96: SPICY ROASTED CHICKPEAS

Prep Time: 35 minutes
Servings: 4
Cooking Method: Oven
Nutritional Values:

- Calories: 120 per serving
- Protein: 5g
- Carbohydrates: 18g
- Fat: 4g

Difficulty: 2/5

Ingredients:

- 1 can (15 oz) chickpeas, drained and rinsed
- 1 tbsp olive oil
- 1 tsp chili powder
- 1/2 tsp cumin
- 1/2 tsp paprika
- Salt to taste

Procedure:

- Preheat oven to 400°F (200°C).
- Pat chickpeas dry with a paper towel.
- Toss chickpeas with olive oil, chili powder, cumin, paprika, and salt.
- Spread evenly on a baking sheet.
- Roast for 25-30 minutes, stirring occasionally, until crispy.

RECIPE 97: APPLE SLICES WITH ALMOND BUTTER

Prep Time: 5 minutes
Servings: 1
Cooking Method: No cooking required
Nutritional Values:

- Calories: 180 per serving
- Protein: 4g
- Carbohydrates: 24g
- Fat: 8g

Difficulty: 1/5

Ingredients:

- 1 apple, sliced
- 2 tbsp almond butter

Procedure:

- Slice the apple into wedges.
- Serve with almond butter for dipping.

RECIPE 98: GREEK YOGURT WITH BERRIES

Prep Time: 5 minutes
Servings: 1
Cooking Method: No cooking required
Nutritional Values:

- Calories: 200 per serving
- Protein: 14g
- Carbohydrates: 25g
- Fat: 5g

Difficulty: 1/5

Ingredients:

- 1 cup Greek yogurt
- 1/2 cup mixed berries (strawberries, blueberries, raspberries)
- 1 tbsp honey

Procedure:

- Spoon Greek yogurt into a bowl.
- Top with mixed berries.
- Drizzle with honey.

RECIPE 99: VEGGIE STICKS WITH HUMMUS

Prep Time: 10 minutes
Servings: 1
Cooking Method: No cooking required
Nutritional Values:

- Calories: 150 per serving
- Protein: 4g
- Carbohydrates: 18g
- Fat: 8g

Difficulty: 1/5

Ingredients:
1/2 cup carrot sticks
1/2 cup celery sticks
1/2 cup bell pepper strips
1/2 cup hummus

Procedure:

- Slice vegetables into sticks.
- Serve with hummus for dipping.

RECIPE 100: DARK CHOCOLATE AND NUT CLUSTERS

Prep Time: 15 minutes
Servings: 12 clusters
Cooking Method: No cooking required
Nutritional Values:

- Calories: 100 per cluster
- Protein: 2g
- Carbohydrates: 10g
- Fat: 7g

Difficulty: 2/5

Ingredients:

- 1 cup dark chocolate chips
- 1/2 cup mixed nuts (almonds, walnuts, pecans)

Procedure:

- Melt dark chocolate chips in a microwave-safe bowl in 30-second intervals, stirring in between, until smooth.
- Stir in mixed nuts.
- Drop spoonfuls of the mixture onto a baking sheet lined with parchment paper.
- Refrigerate until set, about 30 minutes.

RECIPE 101: TURMERIC-SPICED NUTS

Prep Time: 10 minutes
Servings: 4
Cooking Method: Stovetop
Nutritional Values:

- Calories: 200 per serving
- Protein: 5g
- Carbohydrates: 6g
- Fat: 18g

Difficulty: 2/5

Ingredients:

- 1 cup mixed nuts (almonds, cashews, walnuts)
- 1 tbsp olive oil
- 1/2 tsp ground turmeric
- 1/4 tsp ground black pepper
- 1/4 tsp sea salt

Procedure:

- Heat olive oil in a skillet over medium heat.
- Add mixed nuts and stir to coat with oil.
- Sprinkle turmeric, black pepper, and sea salt over the nuts.
- Cook, stirring frequently, for about 5-7 minutes until nuts are golden and fragrant.
- Remove from heat and let cool before serving.

RECIPE 102: CUCUMBER AVOCADO BITES

Prep Time: 10 minutes
Servings: 2
Cooking Method: No cooking required
Nutritional Values:

- Calories: 150 per serving
- Protein: 2g
- Carbohydrates: 12g
- Fat: 11g

Difficulty: 1/5

Ingredients:
1 cucumber, sliced
1 avocado, mashed
1 tbsp lime juice
1 tbsp chopped cilantro
Salt and pepper to taste

Procedure:

- In a small bowl, mash avocado with lime juice, cilantro, salt, and pepper.
- Spread a spoonful of the avocado mixture on each cucumber slice.
- Serve immediately.

RECIPE 103: SWEET POTATO TOAST

Prep Time: 20 minutes
Servings: 2
Cooking Method: Oven
Nutritional Values:

- Calories: 180 per serving
- Protein: 2g
- Carbohydrates: 25g
- Fat: 9g

Difficulty: 2/5

Ingredients:

- 1 medium sweet potato, sliced lengthwise into 1/4-inch slices
- 1 tbsp olive oil
- 1/2 avocado, sliced
- 1 tbsp chia seeds
- Salt and pepper to taste

Procedure:

- Preheat oven to 400°F (200°C).
- Brush sweet potato slices with olive oil and place on a baking sheet.
- Bake for 15 minutes, or until tender.
- Top each slice with avocado, chia seeds, salt, and pepper.
- Serve warm.

RECIPE 104: BLUEBERRY CHIA SEED JAM WITH CRACKERS

Prep Time: 10 minutes (plus cooling time)
Servings: 4
Cooking Method: Stovetop
Nutritional Values:

- Calories: 120 per serving
- Protein: 2g
- Carbohydrates: 20g
- Fat: 4g

Difficulty: 2/5

Ingredients:

- 1 cup fresh blueberries
- 2 tbsp chia seeds
- 1 tbsp honey
- 1 tsp lemon juice
- Whole grain crackers

Procedure:

- In a small saucepan, combine blueberries, chia seeds, honey, and lemon juice.
- Cook over medium heat, stirring occasionally, until blueberries break down and mixture thickens, about 5 minutes.
- Remove from heat and let cool.
- Serve with whole grain crackers.

Prep Time: 5 minutes
Servings: 2
Cooking Method: Stovetop
Nutritional Values:

- Calories: 90 per serving
- Protein: 8g
- Carbohydrates: 8g
- Fat: 3g

Difficulty: 1/5

Ingredients:

- 1 cup shelled edamame (soybeans)
- 1 tsp sea salt

Procedure:

- Bring a pot of water to a boil.
- Add shelled edamame and cook for 3-5 minutes until tender.
- Drain and sprinkle with sea salt.
- Serve warm or chilled.

DESSERTS

RECIPE 106: DARK CHOCOLATE AVOCADO MOUSSE

Prep Time: 10 minutes
Servings: 2
Cooking Method: No cooking required
Nutritional Values:

- Calories: 200 per serving
- Protein: 3g
- Carbohydrates: 25g
- Fat: 12g

Difficulty: 1/5

Ingredients:

- 1 ripe avocado
- 1/4 cup cocoa powder
- 1/4 cup maple syrup
- 1 tsp vanilla extract
- Pinch of sea salt

Procedure:

- Blend avocado, cocoa powder, maple syrup, vanilla extract, and sea salt until smooth.
- Spoon the mousse into small bowls or ramekins.
- Chill in the refrigerator for at least 30 minutes before serving.

RECIPE 107: CHIA SEED PUDDING WITH COCONUT MILK

Prep Time: 5 minutes (plus overnight chilling)
Servings: 2
Cooking Method: No cooking required
Nutritional Values:

- Calories: 180 per serving
- Protein: 4g
- Carbohydrates: 15g
- Fat: 12g

Difficulty: 1/5

Ingredients:

- 1/4 cup chia seeds
- 1 cup coconut milk
- 1 tbsp honey
- 1/2 tsp vanilla extract

Procedure:

- In a bowl, mix chia seeds, coconut milk, honey, and vanilla extract.
- Stir well and refrigerate overnight.
- Stir again before serving and top with fresh fruit if desired.

RECIPE 108: BAKED APPLES WITH CINNAMON

Prep Time: 10 minutes
Servings: 2
Cooking Method: Oven
Nutritional Values:

- Calories: 150 per serving
- Protein: 2g
- Carbohydrates: 28g
- Fat: 6g

Difficulty: 2/5

Ingredients:

- 2 large apples
- 1 tbsp maple syrup
- 1 tsp ground cinnamon
- 1/4 cup chopped walnuts

Procedure:

- Preheat oven to 350°F (175°C).
- Core apples and place them in a baking dish.
- Drizzle with maple syrup, sprinkle with cinnamon, and top with walnuts.
- Bake for 25-30 minutes until tender.

RECIPE 109: ALMOND FLOUR BROWNIES

Prep Time: 15 minutes
Servings: 8
Cooking Method: Oven
Nutritional Values:

- Calories: 190 per serving
- Protein: 4g
- Carbohydrates: 10g
- Fat: 15g

Difficulty: 3/5

Ingredients:

- 1 cup almond flour
- 1/2 cup cocoa powder
- 1/4 tsp sea salt
- 1/4 tsp baking soda
- 1/4 cup coconut oil, melted
- 1/4 cup maple syrup
- 2 large eggs
- 1 tsp vanilla extract

Procedure:

- Preheat oven to 350°F (175°C).
- In a bowl, combine almond flour, cocoa powder, sea salt, and baking soda.
- In another bowl, mix melted coconut oil, maple syrup, eggs, and vanilla extract.
- Combine the wet and dry ingredients and stir until well mixed.
- Pour batter into a greased baking dish and bake for 20-25 minutes.

RECIPE 110: COCONUT MACAROONS

Prep Time: 10 minutes
Servings: 12
Cooking Method: Oven
Nutritional Values:

- Calories: 90 per serving
- Protein: 1g
- Carbohydrates: 8g
- Fat: 7g

Difficulty: 2/5

Ingredients:

- 2 cups shredded coconut
- 1/4 cup honey
- 2 large egg whites
- 1/2 tsp vanilla extract

Procedure:

- Preheat oven to 350°F (175°C).
- In a bowl, mix shredded coconut, honey, egg whites, and vanilla extract.
- Scoop small mounds onto a baking sheet lined with parchment paper.
- Bake for 15-20 minutes until golden.

RECIPE 111: BERRY YOGURT PARFAIT

Prep Time: 5 minutes
Servings: 1
Cooking Method: No cooking required
Nutritional Values:

- Calories: 200 per serving
- Protein: 10g
- Carbohydrates: 25g
- Fat: 5g

Difficulty: 1/5

Ingredients:

- 1 cup Greek yogurt
- 1/2 cup mixed berries (blueberries, strawberries, raspberries)
- 1 tbsp honey
- 1 tbsp chia seeds

Procedure:

- Layer Greek yogurt, mixed berries, and honey in a glass or bowl.
- Sprinkle with chia seeds.
- Serve immediately.

RECIPE 112: QUINOA FRUIT SALAD

Prep Time: 20 minutes
Servings: 2
Cooking Method: No cooking required
Nutritional Values:

- Calories: 180 per serving
- Protein: 4g
- Carbohydrates: 40g
- Fat: 2g

Difficulty: 1/5

Ingredients:

- 1 cup cooked quinoa
- 1/2 cup diced mango
- 1/2 cup diced pineapple
- 1/2 cup blueberries
- 2 tbsp lime juice
- 1 tbsp honey
- 1 tbsp chopped mint

Procedure:

- In a bowl, combine cooked quinoa, diced mango, pineapple, and blueberries.
- In a small bowl, mix lime juice, honey, and chopped mint.
- Drizzle the dressing over the fruit and quinoa mixture.
- Toss gently to combine and serve chilled.

RECIPE 113: LEMON CHIA SEED COOKIES

Prep Time: 15 minutes
Servings: 12
Cooking Method: Oven
Nutritional Values:

- Calories: 120 per serving
- Protein: 2g
- Carbohydrates: 10g
- Fat: 8g

Difficulty: 2/5

Ingredients:

- 1 cup almond flour
- 1/4 cup coconut flour
- 1/4 cup honey
- 2 tbsp chia seeds
- 1 tbsp lemon zest
- 1/4 cup coconut oil, melted
- 1 large egg
- 1/2 tsp baking soda

Procedure:

- Preheat oven to 350°F (175°C).
- In a bowl, mix almond flour, coconut flour, chia seeds, lemon zest, and baking soda.
- In another bowl, combine honey, melted coconut oil, and egg.
- Mix the wet ingredients into the dry ingredients until a dough forms.
- Scoop dough onto a baking sheet lined with parchment paper and flatten slightly.
- Bake for 10-12 minutes until golden.

RECIPE 114: MANGO COCONUT SORBET

Prep Time: 5 minutes (plus freezing time)
Servings: 2
Cooking Method: Freezer
Nutritional Values:

- Calories: 150 per serving
- Protein: 1g
- Carbohydrates: 35g
- Fat: 3g

Difficulty: 1/5

Ingredients:

- 2 ripe mangoes, peeled and chopped
- 1/2 cup coconut milk
- 1 tbsp lime juice

Procedure:

- Blend chopped mangoes, coconut milk, and lime juice until smooth.
- Pour the mixture into a freezer-safe container and freeze for at least 2 hours.
- Scoop and serve.

RECIPE 115: BANANA OAT COOKIES

Prep Time: 10 minutes
Servings: 8
Cooking Method: Oven
Nutritional Values:

- Calories: 80 per serving
- Protein: 2g
- Carbohydrates: 18g
- Fat: 1g

Difficulty: 1/5

Ingredients:

- 2 ripe bananas, mashed
- 1 cup rolled oats
- 1/4 cup raisins
- 1 tsp cinnamon

Procedure:

- Preheat oven to 350°F (175°C).
- In a bowl, mix mashed bananas, rolled oats, raisins, and cinnamon.
- Drop spoonfuls of the mixture onto a baking sheet lined with parchment paper.
- Bake for 15-20 minutes until golden.

RECIPE 116: RASPBERRY CHIA SEED JAM

Prep Time: 10 minutes (plus cooling time)
Servings: 4
Cooking Method: Stovetop
Nutritional Values:

- Calories: 60 per serving
- Protein: 1g
- Carbohydrates: 10g
- Fat: 2g

Difficulty: 1/5

Ingredients:

- 1 cup fresh raspberries
- 2 tbsp chia seeds
- 1 tbsp honey
- 1 tsp lemon juice

Procedure:

- In a small saucepan, combine raspberries, chia seeds, honey, and lemon juice.
- Cook over medium heat, stirring occasionally, until raspberries break down and mixture thickens, about 5 minutes.
- Remove from heat and let cool.
- Serve with whole grain crackers.

RECIPE 117: CARROT CAKE ENERGY BITES

Prep Time: 15 minutes
Servings: 12
Cooking Method: No cooking required
Nutritional Values:

- Calories: 90 per serving
- Protein: 2g
- Carbohydrates: 10g
- Fat: 5g

Difficulty: 2/5

Ingredients:

- 1 cup shredded carrots
- 1 cup rolled oats
- 1/2 cup almond butter
- 1/4 cup honey
- 1/4 cup shredded coconut
- 1 tsp cinnamon
- 1/2 tsp nutmeg

Procedure:

- In a large bowl, mix shredded carrots, rolled oats, almond butter, honey, shredded coconut, cinnamon, and nutmeg until well combined.
- Roll mixture into small balls and place on a baking sheet lined with parchment paper.
- Refrigerate for at least 30 minutes before serving.

RECIPE 118: PINEAPPLE COCONUT BARS

Prep Time: 20 minutes
Servings: 8
Cooking Method: Oven
Nutritional Values:

- Calories: 160 per serving
- Protein: 2g
- Carbohydrates: 20g
- Fat: 8g

Difficulty: 3/5

Ingredients:

- 1 cup crushed pineapple, drained
- 1 cup shredded coconut
- 1/4 cup honey
- 1/4 cup almond flour
- 1/4 cup coconut oil, melted
- 1 tsp vanilla extract

Procedure:

- Preheat oven to 350°F (175°C).
- In a bowl, mix crushed pineapple, shredded coconut, honey, almond flour, melted coconut oil, and vanilla extract until well combined.
- Press mixture into a baking dish lined with parchment paper.
- Bake for 25-30 minutes until golden.
- Let cool before cutting into bars.

RECIPE 119: MATCHA GREEN TEA ICE CREAM

Prep Time: 10 minutes (plus freezing time)
Servings: 2
Cooking Method: Freezer
Nutritional Values:

- Calories: 150 per serving
- Protein: 1g
- Carbohydrates: 25g
- Fat: 6g

Difficulty: 2/5

Ingredients:

- 1 cup coconut milk
- 1 tbsp matcha green tea powder
- 1/4 cup honey
- 1 tsp vanilla extract

Procedure:

- In a bowl, whisk together coconut milk, matcha green tea powder, honey, and vanilla extract until smooth.
- Pour the mixture into an ice cream maker and churn according to the manufacturer's instructions.
- Transfer to a freezer-safe container and freeze for at least 2 hours before serving.

Prep Time: 15 minutes
Servings: 2
Cooking Method: Microwave
Nutritional Values:

- Calories: 100 per serving
- Protein: 1g
- Carbohydrates: 15g
- Fat: 6g

Difficulty: 1/5

Ingredients:

- 1 cup fresh strawberries
- 1/2 cup dark chocolate chips
- 1 tbsp coconut oil

Procedure:

- Wash and dry the strawberries.
- In a microwave-safe bowl, combine dark chocolate chips and coconut oil.
- Microwave in 30-second intervals, stirring until melted and smooth.
- Dip each strawberry into the melted chocolate, coating evenly.
- Place on a parchment-lined baking sheet and refrigerate until chocolate is set.

ANTI-INFLAMMATORY SMOOTHIES AND JUICES

RECIPE 121: TROPICAL TURMERIC SMOOTHIE

Prep Time: 5 minutes
Servings: 1
Cooking Method: Blender
Nutritional Values:

- Calories: 200
- Protein: 2g
- Carbohydrates: 50g
- Fat: 1g

Difficulty: 1/5

Ingredients:

- 1 cup coconut water
- 1/2 cup frozen pineapple chunks
- 1/2 cup frozen mango chunks
- 1 banana
- 1 tsp turmeric powder
- 1/2 tsp ground ginger

Procedure:

- Combine all ingredients in a blender.
- Blend until smooth.
- Pour into a glass and serve immediately.

RECIPE 122: BERRY BEET JUICE

Prep Time: 10 minutes
Servings: 1
Cooking Method: Juicer
Nutritional Values:

- Calories: 150
- Protein: 2g
- Carbohydrates: 35g
- Fat: 0g

Difficulty: 2/5

Ingredients:

- 1 medium beet, peeled and chopped
- 1 cup strawberries
- 1/2 cup blueberries
- 1 apple, cored and chopped
- 1/2 lemon, juiced

Procedure:

- Run the beet, strawberries, blueberries, and apple through a juicer.
- Stir in the lemon juice.
- Pour into a glass and serve immediately.

RECIPE 123: GREEN DETOX SMOOTHIE

Prep Time: 5 minutes

Ingredients:

Servings: 1
Cooking Method: Blender
Nutritional Values:

- Calories: 250
- Protein: 5g
- Carbohydrates: 30g
- Fat: 15g

Difficulty: 1/5

- 1 cup spinach
- 1/2 cup cucumber, chopped
- 1/2 green apple, chopped
- 1/2 avocado
- 1 cup almond milk
- 1 tbsp chia seeds

Procedure:

- Combine all ingredients in a blender.
- Blend until smooth.
- Pour into a glass and serve immediately.

RECIPE 124: GINGER CARROT JUICE

Prep Time: 10 minutes
Servings: 1
Cooking Method: Juicer
Nutritional Values:

- Calories: 120
- Protein: 2g
- Carbohydrates: 30g
- Fat: 0g

Difficulty: 2/5

Ingredients:

- 4 large carrots, peeled
- 1 inch fresh ginger, peeled
- 1 orange, peeled
- 1/2 lemon, juiced

Procedure:

- Run the carrots, ginger, and orange through a juicer.
- Stir in the lemon juice.
- Pour into a glass and serve immediately.

RECIPE 125: ANTI-INFLAMMATORY GOLDEN MILK SMOOTHIE

Prep Time: 5 minutes
Servings: 1
Cooking Method: Blender
Nutritional Values:

- Calories: 130
- Protein: 2g
- Carbohydrates: 28g

Ingredients:

- 1 cup unsweetened almond milk
- 1/2 banana
- 1/2 tsp turmeric powder
- 1/4 tsp cinnamon
- 1/2 tsp ginger powder
- 1 tsp honey

- Fat: 3g

Difficulty: 1/5

Procedure:

- Combine all ingredients in a blender.
- Blend until smooth.
- Pour into a glass and serve immediately.

RECIPE 126: PINEAPPLE GREEN JUICE

Prep Time: 10 minutes
Servings: 1
Cooking Method: Juicer
Nutritional Values:

- Calories: 100
- Protein: 1g
- Carbohydrates: 24g
- Fat: 0g

Difficulty: 2/5

Ingredients:

- 1 cup pineapple chunks
- 1/2 cucumber, chopped
- 1 cup spinach
- 1/2 lime, juiced
- 1 inch fresh ginger, peeled

Procedure:

- Run the pineapple, cucumber, spinach, and ginger through a juicer.
- Stir in the lime juice.
- Pour into a glass and serve immediately.

RECIPE 127: BLUEBERRY KALE SMOOTHIE

Prep Time: 5 minutes
Servings: 1
Cooking Method: Blender
Nutritional Values:

- Calories: 150
- Protein: 3g
- Carbohydrates: 35g
- Fat: 2g

Difficulty: 1/5

Ingredients:

- 1 cup kale leaves
- 1/2 cup frozen blueberries
- 1/2 banana
- 1 cup coconut water
- 1 tbsp flaxseeds

Procedure:

- Combine all ingredients in a blender.
- Blend until smooth.

- Pour into a glass and serve immediately.

RECIPE 128: SPICY TOMATO JUICE

Prep Time: 10 minutes
Servings: 1
Cooking Method: Juicer
Nutritional Values:

- Calories: 80
- Protein: 3g
- Carbohydrates: 18g
- Fat: 0g

Difficulty: 2/5

Ingredients:

- 4 large tomatoes, chopped
- 1 celery stalk, chopped
- 1/2 cucumber, chopped
- 1/4 tsp cayenne pepper
- 1/2 lemon, juiced

Procedure:

- Run the tomatoes, celery, and cucumber through a juicer.
- Stir in the cayenne pepper and lemon juice.
- Pour into a glass and serve immediately.

RECIPE 129: APPLE CINNAMON SMOOTHIE

Prep Time: 5 minutes
Servings: 1
Cooking Method: Blender
Nutritional Values:

- Calories: 200
- Protein: 8g
- Carbohydrates: 35g
- Fat: 5g

Difficulty: 1/5

Ingredients:

- 1 apple, chopped
- 1/2 banana
- 1/2 cup Greek yogurt
- 1/2 tsp cinnamon
- 1 cup almond milk

Procedure:

- Combine all ingredients in a blender.
- Blend until smooth.
- Pour into a glass and serve immediately.

RECIPE 130: TROPICAL GREEN JUICE

Prep Time: 10 minutes
Servings: 1
Cooking Method: Juicer
Nutritional Values:

- Calories: 90
- Protein: 2g
- Carbohydrates: 20g
- Fat: 1g

Difficulty: 2/5

Ingredients:

- 1 cup kale leaves
- 1/2 cup pineapple chunks
- 1/2 cucumber, chopped
- 1/2 lemon, juiced
- 1 inch fresh ginger, peeled

Procedure:

- Run the kale, pineapple, cucumber, and ginger through a juicer.
- Stir in the lemon juice.
- Pour into a glass and serve immediately.

RECIPE 131: WATERMELON MINT JUICE

Prep Time: 5 minutes
Servings: 1
Cooking Method: Blender
Nutritional Values:

- Calories: 80
- Protein: 1g
- Carbohydrates: 20g
- Fat: 0g

Difficulty: 1/5

Ingredients:

- 2 cups watermelon, chopped
- 1/4 cup fresh mint leaves
- 1/2 lime, juiced

Procedure:

- Combine all ingredients in a blender.
- Blend until smooth.
- Pour into a glass and serve immediately.

RECIPE 132: CITRUS GREEN TEA SMOOTHIE

Prep Time: 5 minutes
Servings: 1
Cooking Method: Blender
Nutritional Values:

Ingredients:

- 1 cup brewed green tea, cooled
- 1 orange, peeled and chopped
- 1/2 banana

- Calories: 150
- Protein: 2g
- Carbohydrates: 35g
- Fat: 1g

- 1/2 cup spinach
- 1 tbsp honey

Difficulty: 1/5

Procedure:

- Combine all ingredients in a blender.
- Blend until smooth.
- Pour into a glass and serve immediately.

RECIPE 133: GINGER LEMONADE

Prep Time: 5 minutes
Servings: 1
Cooking Method: Stovetop
Nutritional Values:

- Calories: 60
- Protein: 0g
- Carbohydrates: 15g
- Fat: 0g

Ingredients:

- 1 cup water
- 1 lemon, juiced
- 1 inch fresh ginger, peeled and grated
- 1 tbsp honey

Difficulty: 1/5

Procedure:

- Heat water in a saucepan until warm.
- Add lemon juice, grated ginger, and honey. Stir well.
- Pour into a glass and serve warm.

RECIPE 134: SPICED APPLE CIDER

Prep Time: 10 minutes
Servings: 1
Cooking Method: Stovetop
Nutritional Values:

- Calories: 120
- Protein: 0g
- Carbohydrates: 30g
- Fat: 0g

Ingredients:

- 1 cup apple cider
- 1 cinnamon stick
- 1/4 tsp ground cloves
- 1/4 tsp ground nutmeg

Difficulty: 1/5

Procedure:

- In a small saucepan, combine apple cider, cinnamon stick, ground cloves, and ground nutmeg.
- Heat over medium heat until warm.
- Pour into a mug and serve.

RECIPE 135: BERRY CHIA SEED JUICE

Prep Time: 10 minutes
Servings: 1
Cooking Method: Blender
Nutritional Values:

- Calories: 100
- Protein: 2g
- Carbohydrates: 25g
- Fat: 1g

Difficulty: 1/5

Ingredients:

- 1 cup mixed berries (strawberries, blueberries, raspberries)
- 1 cup water
- 1 tbsp chia seeds
- 1 tbsp honey

Procedure:

- Combine mixed berries, water, chia seeds, and honey in a blender.
- Blend until smooth.
- Pour into a glass and let sit for 5 minutes to allow chia seeds to expand.
- Serve and enjoy.

TEAS AND BEVERAGES

RECIPE 136: GINGER TURMERIC TEA

Prep Time: 10 minutes
Servings: 2
Cooking Method: Stovetop
Nutritional Values:

- Calories: 45
- Protein: 0g
- Carbohydrates: 12g
- Fat: 0g

Difficulty: 1/5

Ingredients:

- 1 inch fresh ginger, peeled and sliced
- 1 tsp turmeric powder
- 1 tbsp honey
- 2 cups water
- 1 lemon, sliced

Procedure:

- In a small saucepan, bring water to a boil.
- Add sliced ginger and turmeric powder.
- Reduce heat and simmer for 5 minutes.
- Strain into cups, add honey and lemon slices, stir well and serve hot.

RECIPE 137: CHAMOMILE LAVENDER TEA

Prep Time: 5 minutes
Servings: 2
Cooking Method: Steeping
Nutritional Values:

- Calories: 5
- Protein: 0g
- Carbohydrates: 1g
- Fat: 0g

Difficulty: 1/5

Ingredients:

- 2 tsp dried chamomile flowers
- 1 tsp dried lavender flowers
- 2 cups boiling water
- 1 tsp honey (optional)

Procedure:

- Place chamomile and lavender flowers in a teapot.
- Pour boiling water over the flowers.
- Let steep for 5 minutes.
- Strain into cups, add honey if desired.
- Serve hot.

RECIPE 138: MINT GREEN TEA

Prep Time: 5 minutes
Servings: 2
Cooking Method: Steeping
Nutritional Values:

- Calories: 20
- Protein: 0g
- Carbohydrates: 5g
- Fat: 0g

Difficulty: 1/5

Ingredients:

- 1 green tea bag
- 1/4 cup fresh mint leaves
- 2 cups boiling water
- 1 tsp honey

Procedure:

- Place green tea bag and mint leaves in a teapot.
- Pour boiling water over the tea and mint.
- Let steep for 3 minutes.
- Strain into cups, add honey.
- Serve hot.

RECIPE 139: SPICED APPLE CIDER

Prep Time: 10 minutes
Servings: 2
Cooking Method: Stovetop
Nutritional Values:

- Calories: 120
- Protein: 0g
- Carbohydrates: 30g
- Fat: 0g

Difficulty: 2/5

Ingredients:

- 2 cups apple cider
- 1 cinnamon stick
- 3 cloves
- 1/4 tsp ground nutmeg
- 1 orange, sliced

Procedure:

- In a small saucepan, combine apple cider, cinnamon stick, cloves, and nutmeg.
- Heat over medium heat until warm.
- Add orange slices and simmer for 5 minutes.
- Strain into cups and serve hot.

RECIPE 140: LEMON GINGER DETOX WATER

Prep Time: 5 minutes
Servings: 4
Cooking Method: None
Nutritional Values:

- Calories: 5
- Protein: 0g
- Carbohydrates: 1g
- Fat: 0g

Difficulty: 1/5

Ingredients:

- 1 lemon, sliced
- 1 inch fresh ginger, peeled and sliced
- 1 cucumber, sliced
- 8 cups water

Procedure:

- Combine lemon, ginger, cucumber, and water in a large pitcher.
- Refrigerate for at least 1 hour.
- Serve chilled.

RECIPE 141: GOLDEN MILK

Prep Time: 5 minutes
Servings: 1
Cooking Method: Stovetop
Nutritional Values:

- Calories: 70
- Protein: 1g
- Carbohydrates: 12g
- Fat: 2g

Difficulty: 1/5

Ingredients:

- 1 cup unsweetened almond milk
- 1/2 tsp turmeric powder
- 1/4 tsp cinnamon
- 1/4 tsp ginger powder
- 1 tsp honey
- Pinch of black pepper

Procedure:

- Heat almond milk in a small saucepan over medium heat.
- Add turmeric, cinnamon, ginger, honey, and black pepper.
- Stir well and bring to a simmer.
- Pour into a cup and serve hot.

RECIPE 142: HIBISCUS ICED TEA

Prep Time: 10 minutes
Servings: 4
Cooking Method: Stovetop
Nutritional Values:

- Calories: 60
- Protein: 0g
- Carbohydrates: 16g
- Fat: 0g

Difficulty: 1/5

Ingredients:

- 1/4 cup dried hibiscus flowers
- 4 cups water
- 1/4 cup honey
- 1/4 cup lime juice

Procedure:

- Bring water to a boil in a medium pot.
- Remove from heat and add hibiscus flowers.
- Let steep for 10 minutes.
- Strain into a pitcher and stir in honey and lime juice.
- Refrigerate until chilled and serve over ice.

RECIPE 143: MATCHA LATTE

Prep Time: 5 minutes
Servings: 1
Cooking Method: Stovetop
Nutritional Values:

- Calories: 60
- Protein: 1g
- Carbohydrates: 12g
- Fat: 2g

Difficulty: 1/5

Ingredients:

- 1 tsp matcha powder
- 1 cup unsweetened almond milk
- 1 tsp honey
- 1/4 tsp vanilla extract

Procedure:

- Heat almond milk in a small saucepan over medium heat.
- In a mug, whisk matcha powder with a small amount of hot almond milk until smooth.
- Add honey and vanilla extract, then pour in the remaining almond milk.
- Stir well and serve hot.

RECIPE 144: CINNAMON SPICED TEA

Prep Time: 10 minutes
Servings: 2
Cooking Method: Stovetop
Nutritional Values:

- Calories: 30
- Protein: 0g
- Carbohydrates: 8g
- Fat: 0g

Difficulty: 1/5

Ingredients:

- 2 cups water
- 1 cinnamon stick
- 2 black tea bags
- 1/2 tsp ground cinnamon
- 1 tsp honey

Procedure:

- Bring water and cinnamon stick to a boil in a small saucepan.
- Remove from heat and add tea bags.
- Steep for 5 minutes.
- Remove tea bags and cinnamon stick.
- Stir in ground cinnamon and honey.
- Pour into cups and serve hot.

RECIPE 145: COCONUT LIME WATER

Prep Time: 5 minutes
Servings: 1
Cooking Method: None
Nutritional Values:

- Calories: 60
- Protein: 0g
- Carbohydrates: 16g
- Fat: 0g

Difficulty: 1/5

Ingredients:

- 1 cup coconut water
- 1/2 lime, juiced
- 1 tbsp honey
- Ice cubes

Procedure:

- In a glass, combine coconut water, lime juice, and honey.
- Stir well until honey is dissolved.
- Add ice cubes and serve chilled.

RECIPE 146: BLUEBERRY MINT COOLER

Prep Time: 5 minutes
Servings: 2
Cooking Method: None
Nutritional Values:

- Calories: 40
- Protein: 0g
- Carbohydrates: 10g
- Fat: 0g

Difficulty: 1/5

Ingredients:

- 1/2 cup blueberries
- 1/4 cup fresh mint leaves
- 1 tbsp honey
- 2 cups sparkling water
- Ice cubes

Procedure:

- In a pitcher, combine blueberries and mint leaves.
- Muddle the ingredients to release their flavors.
- Add honey and sparkling water.
- Stir well and pour over ice cubes in glasses.
- Serve immediately.

RECIPE 147: ROSEHIP HIBISCUS TEA

Prep Time: 10 minutes
Servings: 2
Cooking Method: Steeping
Nutritional Values:

- Calories: 30
- Protein: 0g
- Carbohydrates: 8g
- Fat: 0g

Difficulty: 1/5

Ingredients:

- 2 tbsp dried rosehip
- 1 tbsp dried hibiscus flowers
- 2 cups boiling water
- 1 tsp honey

Procedure:

- Combine dried rosehip and hibiscus flowers in a teapot.
- Pour boiling water over the dried ingredients.
- Let steep for 10 minutes.
- Strain into cups and stir in honey.
- Serve hot.

Conclusion

Adopting a new way of eating focused on reducing inflammation can significantly improve your quality of life. The recipes in this chapter provide a practical and enjoyable way to start this journey. By incorporating more fresh vegetables, fruits, lean proteins, and healthy fats into your meals, you can support your body's natural ability to heal and manage the symptoms of fibromyalgia.

Consistency is key. While it may take time for your body to adjust to the new dietary habits, the benefits will become evident as inflammation decreases and energy levels improve. Don't be discouraged by the occasional craving for processed foods or dairy; instead, remember the long-term goals of better health and reduced symptoms.

If necessary, supplement your diet with specific nutrients to ensure you're meeting all your nutritional needs. For example, omega-3 fatty acids, vitamin D, and magnesium are known to help reduce inflammation and support overall health. Consult with a healthcare professional to determine the best supplements for your individual needs.

By committing to these dietary changes, you are taking a powerful step toward managing fibromyalgia and improving your overall well-being. Enjoy the journey and the delicious, healthful meals along the way.

SUMMARY TABLE: FOODS TO EAT VS. FOODS TO AVOID

Foods to Eat	Foods to Avoid
Fresh vegetables	Processed foods
Fruits	Sugary drinks
Lean proteins	Red meat and processed meats
Whole grains	Refined grains
Healthy fats	Trans fats
Nuts and seeds	Dairy products
Anti-inflammatory spices	Artificial sweeteners and additives
Herbal teas and water	Alcohol and caffeinated beverages

Fresh vegetables (e.g., leafy greens, broccoli, carrots, spinach, kale, bell peppers, zucchini, tomatoes, cucumbers, cauliflower)

Fruits (e.g., berries, citrus, apples, pears, bananas, mangoes, pineapples, grapes, kiwi, peaches)

Lean proteins (e.g., chicken, fish, turkey, tofu, tempeh, eggs, lentils, beans, Greek yogurt, chickpeas)

Whole grains (e.g., quinoa, brown rice, oats, barley, whole wheat, farro, bulgur, millet, spelt, buckwheat)

Healthy fats (e.g., olive oil, avocado, coconut oil, flaxseed oil, walnuts, chia seeds, hemp seeds, almonds, fatty fish, dark chocolate)

Nuts and seeds (e.g., almonds, chia, flaxseeds, pumpkin seeds, sunflower seeds, walnuts, pecans, hazelnuts, pistachios, cashews)

Anti-inflammatory spices (e.g., turmeric, ginger, cinnamon, garlic, cayenne pepper, black pepper, cumin, coriander, rosemary, basil)

Herbal teas and water (e.g., chamomile tea, peppermint tea, green tea, rooibos tea, ginger tea, hibiscus tea, dandelion tea, fennel tea, lemon balm tea, nettle tea)

Processed foods (e.g., fast food, snacks, microwave meals, packaged desserts, instant noodles, deli meats, canned soups, frozen pizzas, pre-packaged sauces, chips)

Sugary drinks (e.g., sodas, energy drinks, sweetened iced teas, fruit punches, lemonade, sports drinks, sweetened coffee drinks, flavored milk, tonic water, sweetened coconut water)

Red meat and processed meats (e.g., beef, pork, lamb, bacon, sausages, hot dogs, ham, salami, corned beef, deli meats)

Refined grains (e.g., white bread, pasta, white rice, pastries, muffins, cakes, cookies, pancakes, waffles, crackers)

Trans fats (e.g., margarine, fried foods, baked goods with hydrogenated oils, snack foods, frozen dinners, non-dairy coffee creamers, microwave popcorn, shortening, store-bought pie crusts, fast food fries)

Dairy products (e.g., milk, cheese, yogurt, butter, cream, ice cream, cottage cheese, sour cream, cream cheese, powdered milk)

Artificial sweeteners and additives (e.g., aspartame, sucralose, saccharin, high fructose corn syrup, MSG, artificial colors, artificial flavors, preservatives, emulsifiers, texturizers)

Alcohol and caffeinated beverages (e.g., beer, wine, spirits, cocktails, coffee, black tea, soda with caffeine, energy drinks, pre-workout drinks, caffeinated water)

CONCLUSION TO PART II: MEAL PLANS AND RECIPES

As you conclude Part II: Meal Plans and Recipes, remember that the journey to better health through nutrition is both rewarding and transformative. By embracing the 5-week meal plan and integrating the provided recipes into your daily routine, you are taking significant steps toward reducing inflammation and managing fibromyalgia symptoms. These new habits will become easier and more automatic over time, paving the way for a healthier, more vibrant life.

PART 3: TREATMENTS AND SYMPTOM MANAGEMENT

Living with fibromyalgia presents numerous challenges, from managing chronic pain to dealing with fatigue and emotional stress. For persons afflicted with this illness, knowing and putting into practice efficient therapies and symptom management techniques can significantly improve their quality of life. Part III of this book delves into a comprehensive exploration of various medical, pharmacological, and complementary treatments available for fibromyalgia, aiming to provide a holistic approach to managing symptoms.

In this section, we will cover the most commonly prescribed medications that help alleviate the primary symptoms of fibromyalgia. These first-line medications include pain relievers, antidepressants, and anti-seizure drugs, each playing a role in targeting specific aspects of the condition. We will discuss how these medications work, their potential side effects, and the importance of working closely with healthcare providers to tailor a treatment plan that fits individual needs.

Beyond conventional medicine, the field of alternative and complementary therapies offers a wealth of options that can enhance the overall treatment plan. Techniques such as acupuncture, massage therapy, and the use of supplements and natural remedies can provide significant relief. We will explore these therapies in detail, backed by scientific explanations and research findings that support their effectiveness. Understanding the benefits and limitations of these treatments can empower patients to make informed decisions about incorporating them into their daily routines.

Additionally, we will address the importance of physical exercise and movement in managing fibromyalgia symptoms. Engaging in regular physical activity, including specific exercises designed for fibromyalgia, yoga, and stretching routines, can help reduce pain and improve overall physical function. This part of the book will provide practical tips and guidelines on how to incorporate exercise safely and effectively, emphasizing the role of consistency and gradual progression.

Mental health and emotional well-being are also critical components of managing fibromyalgia. Stress management techniques, relaxation practices, mindfulness, and meditation can significantly impact the overall experience of living with this condition. We will discuss various strategies to enhance mental resilience, reduce anxiety, and promote a positive outlook, recognizing that emotional health is intrinsically linked to physical well-being.

Lastly, sleep hygiene is a vital aspect of symptom management. Poor sleep quality can exacerbate pain and fatigue, making it crucial to establish healthy sleep patterns. We will offer practical tips and natural remedies to improve sleep quality, helping to break the cycle of insomnia and pain commonly associated with fibromyalgia.

By integrating these diverse approaches, this part aims to provide a comprehensive toolkit for managing fibromyalgia symptoms effectively. It emphasizes a personalized approach, recognizing that each individual's experience with fibromyalgia is unique. The goal is to empower readers with knowledge and practical strategies that can be tailored to their specific needs, fostering a proactive and informed approach to managing their condition.

CHAPTER 8: MEDICAL AND PHARMACOLOGICAL TREATMENTS

Navigating the myriad of treatment options for fibromyalgia can feel overwhelming. This chapter is designed to provide you with a comprehensive overview of the medical and pharmacological treatments available, helping you make informed decisions about managing your condition. The treatment landscape for fibromyalgia has evolved significantly over the years, offering a range of options from first-line medications to emerging therapies.

First-line medications typically include antidepressants, anti-seizure drugs, and pain relievers. These medications target different aspects of fibromyalgia, such as pain, fatigue, and mood disturbances. Understanding how these drugs work and their potential side effects is crucial for effective management.

In addition to conventional treatments, there is a growing interest in experimental therapies and new discoveries. Research in this area is ongoing, with scientists exploring innovative approaches to alleviate fibromyalgia symptoms. These include techniques such as transcranial magnetic stimulation (TMS), low-dose naltrexone (LDN), and even the use of cannabinoids. While these treatments may hold promise, it is essential to approach them with caution and under the guidance of a healthcare professional.

Natural remedies and supplements are also commonly used by those with fibromyalgia. While they can offer relief, it is important to consider potential interactions with prescribed medications. Herbal supplements like St. John's Wort, valerian root, and others can interact negatively with pharmaceuticals, making it crucial to consult with your healthcare provider before starting any new treatment regimen.

Finally, understanding the potential side effects and interactions of these treatments is key to managing fibromyalgia safely. This chapter will explore the common side effects associated with first-line medications and how to mitigate them. It will also discuss the importance of a collaborative approach with healthcare providers to tailor treatments to your individual needs.

FIRST-LINE MEDICATIONS

When it comes to managing fibromyalgia, first-line medications play a crucial role in alleviating symptoms and improving quality of life. These medications are often prescribed based on their ability to address specific symptoms such as pain, fatigue, and sleep disturbances, which are commonly experienced by individuals with fibromyalgia.

Antidepressants are one of the primary classes of medications used in the treatment of fibromyalgia. Drugs like *amitriptyline* and *duloxetine* have been shown to help reduce pain and improve sleep quality. These medications work by altering the levels of certain chemicals in the brain, which can help modulate pain perception and enhance mood.

Anticonvulsants, such as *pregabalin* and *gabapentin*, are also frequently prescribed. These medications help to calm nerve activity, which can be beneficial for reducing the widespread pain and sensitivity associated with fibromyalgia. By stabilizing the electrical activity in the brain, anticonvulsants can help diminish the pain signals that are often amplified in people with fibromyalgia.

Pain relievers are another cornerstone of fibromyalgia treatment. Over-the-counter options like *acetaminophen* and *nonsteroidal anti-inflammatory drugs (NSAIDs)* such as *ibuprofen* can provide relief for mild to moderate pain. For more severe pain, doctors might prescribe *tramadol*, a centrally acting pain medication that is typically considered when other treatments have not been effective.

In addition to these, **muscle relaxants** like *cyclobenzaprine* can be used to alleviate muscle stiffness and spasms, which are common in fibromyalgia patients. These medications can also improve sleep quality by reducing nighttime muscle activity, helping individuals achieve more restful sleep.

While these first-line medications can significantly help manage fibromyalgia symptoms, it's important to note that their effectiveness can vary from person to person. Working closely with a healthcare provider to find the right combination and dosage is essential for optimizing treatment outcomes. Regular follow-ups and adjustments may be necessary to ensure the best possible management of the condition.

Incorporating lifestyle changes alongside medication can further enhance the benefits, creating a more comprehensive approach to fibromyalgia management.

NATURAL REMEDIES, EXPERIMENTAL THERAPIES, AND NEW DISCOVERIES

Exploring treatments beyond traditional medications can offer fibromyalgia patients additional avenues for symptom relief and overall well-being. This approach integrates natural remedies, experimental therapies, and recent discoveries in medical research, providing a holistic perspective on managing fibromyalgia.

Natural Remedies: Many individuals with fibromyalgia turn to natural remedies to complement their medical treatments. *Herbal supplements*, such as *turmeric*, *ginger*, and *boswellia*, are popular for their anti-inflammatory properties. Turmeric, for instance, contains curcumin, a compound known for its ability to reduce inflammation and pain. Ginger has similar properties and can be easily incorporated into daily meals or taken as a supplement. Boswellia, often referred to as Indian frankincense, is another powerful anti-inflammatory that has shown promise in reducing pain and improving physical function in chronic conditions.

Magnesium supplements are another natural option worth considering. Magnesium plays a crucial role in muscle and nerve function, and deficiencies in this mineral have been linked to increased pain sensitivity and muscle cramps. Taking magnesium supplements or increasing dietary intake through foods like leafy greens, nuts, and seeds can help alleviate these symptoms.

Acupuncture, an ancient Chinese therapy, involves inserting thin needles into specific points on the body to stimulate energy flow and promote healing. Many fibromyalgia patients report significant pain relief and improved energy levels after regular acupuncture sessions. It's essential to seek treatment from a licensed practitioner to ensure safety and efficacy.

Experimental Therapies: The landscape of fibromyalgia treatment is continually evolving, with new therapies being researched and developed. *Transcranial magnetic stimulation (TMS)* is one such therapy that has garnered attention. TMS uses magnetic fields to stimulate nerve cells in the brain, potentially altering pain perception and reducing symptoms. Early studies suggest that TMS may help improve mood and reduce pain in fibromyalgia patients, although more research is needed to confirm its long-term benefits.

Hyperbaric oxygen therapy (HBOT) is another experimental treatment showing promise. HBOT involves breathing pure oxygen in a pressurized environment, which increases oxygen levels in the blood and tissues. Some studies have found that HBOT can reduce pain and fatigue in fibromyalgia patients, possibly by reducing inflammation and promoting tissue repair.

New Discoveries: Medical research continues to uncover new insights into fibromyalgia, leading to innovative treatments. One recent discovery involves the role of the *gut microbiome* in fibromyalgia. Research suggests that imbalances in gut bacteria may contribute to inflammation and pain sensitivity. **Probiotics and prebiotics**, which promote healthy gut bacteria, are being studied for their potential to improve fibromyalgia symptoms. Consuming probiotic-rich foods like yogurt, kefir, and fermented vegetables, or taking a high-quality probiotic supplement, might support gut health and reduce inflammation.

CBD oil, derived from the hemp plant, has gained popularity as a natural remedy for pain and anxiety. CBD interacts with the body's endocannabinoid system, which regulates various functions, including pain and mood. Some fibromyalgia patients report that CBD oil helps reduce pain and improve sleep without the psychoactive effects associated with THC, another compound found in cannabis.

Consulting Specialists: While exploring these alternative treatments, it is crucial to consult healthcare specialists. They can provide guidance on integrating these therapies into your treatment plan safely and effectively. Self-medication, especially with supplements and alternative therapies, can pose risks, including potential interactions with prescribed medications. A healthcare provider can help tailor these treatments to your specific needs and monitor your progress to ensure optimal outcomes.

SIDE EFFECTS AND INTERACTIONS WITH NATURAL REMEDIES

Understanding the side effects and potential interactions between medications and natural remedies is crucial for managing fibromyalgia effectively. When combining treatments, it's essential to be aware of how they might interact to ensure safety and enhance the benefits.

Side Effects: Every medication, including those commonly prescribed for fibromyalgia, comes with potential side effects. For example, *antidepressants* like amitriptyline or duloxetine can cause dizziness, dry mouth, and weight gain. *Anti-seizure medications* such as pregabalin and gabapentin might lead to drowsiness, edema, and blurred vision. It's important to discuss these side effects with your doctor to weigh the benefits and potential risks of each medication.

Interactions with Natural Remedies: Natural remedies can offer relief from fibromyalgia symptoms, but they are not without risks, especially when combined with prescription medications. For instance, *St. John's Wort*, often used for depression, can interfere with the effectiveness of antidepressants and other drugs, potentially leading to serious side effects. Similarly, *valerian root*, commonly taken for sleep disorders, can amplify the sedative effects of certain medications, causing excessive drowsiness or confusion.

Consulting Specialists: The importance of consulting healthcare specialists cannot be overstated. Self-medication with supplements or alternative therapies can be dangerous, especially without professional guidance. Specialists can help you navigate the complexities of combining treatments, ensuring that you receive the most effective and safe care. They can also monitor your progress and make necessary adjustments to your treatment plan.

Common Interactions: Be cautious of combining *omega-3 supplements* with blood-thinning medications, as this can increase the risk of bleeding. Likewise, *magnesium supplements* can interact with certain antibiotics and muscle relaxants, potentially diminishing their effectiveness. Always inform your healthcare provider about any supplements or natural remedies you are considering or currently using.

Practical Steps: To manage side effects and avoid interactions, keep a detailed list of all medications, supplements, and remedies you are taking. Share this list with every healthcare provider you visit to ensure comprehensive care. Regular blood tests and check-ups can also help detect any adverse effects early, allowing for timely adjustments to your treatment plan.

Safe Practices: When introducing a new treatment, start with the lowest possible dose and gradually increase it, monitoring for any side effects. Maintain open communication with your healthcare providers and report any unusual symptoms immediately. This proactive approach helps in managing fibromyalgia more effectively and reduces the risk of complications.

In conclusion, managing fibromyalgia requires a careful balance of medications and natural remedies. By staying informed about potential side effects and interactions, and by consulting with healthcare specialists, you can develop a treatment plan that maximizes benefits and minimizes risks. Always prioritize your safety and well-being, and never hesitate to seek professional advice when considering new treatments.

Conclusion

Managing fibromyalgia is a complex, multifaceted journey that requires a personalized approach. By understanding the various medical and pharmacological treatments available, you can take proactive steps towards managing your symptoms more effectively. First-line medications such as antidepressants, anti-seizure drugs, and pain relievers form the cornerstone of treatment but should be used with an awareness of their potential side effects.

Emerging therapies and experimental treatments offer new hope for those who have not found relief through conventional methods. However, it is essential to approach these with caution and under medical supervision to ensure safety and efficacy. Natural remedies and supplements can complement traditional treatments, but they also carry the risk of interactions and side effects. Therefore, open communication with your healthcare team is vital in crafting a treatment plan that works best for you.

To make this text more fluid and engaging, consider varying sentence lengths and structures to maintain reader interest. Transition smoothly between topics to enhance the flow of information. Consistently use active voice to create a direct and engaging narrative. Avoid repetition by introducing key concepts clearly and concisely, ensuring the content remains fresh and informative.

In summary, fibromyalgia management is a dynamic process that benefits from a well-rounded understanding of available treatments. By staying informed and maintaining close communication with your healthcare providers, you can navigate this journey with greater confidence and hope. Always prioritize your health and safety, and never hesitate to seek professional advice when exploring new treatment options.

CHAPTER 9: ALTERNATIVE AND COMPLEMENTARY THERAPIES

Living with fibromyalgia often requires a multifaceted approach to manage its diverse and chronic symptoms. While conventional medical treatments are a cornerstone of fibromyalgia management, many patients find additional relief through alternative and complementary therapies. These therapies offer a holistic approach, addressing not just the physical aspects of fibromyalgia but also the emotional and psychological well-being of the patient.

Alternative therapies such as acupuncture, massage, and biofeedback have gained popularity for their potential to alleviate pain and improve quality of life. Acupuncture, for example, has roots in traditional Chinese medicine and is increasingly backed by scientific studies demonstrating its ability to reduce pain and enhance overall wellness. Similarly, massage therapy, with its various techniques, can help decrease muscle tension and promote relaxation, significantly benefiting those with fibromyalgia.

In addition to these therapies, practices like Tai Chi and yoga combine physical activity with mindfulness, offering a dual benefit of physical relief and mental relaxation. These practices are particularly valuable for fibromyalgia patients due to their low-impact nature and ability to improve both physical function and emotional health. Supplements and natural remedies also play a role, providing nutritional support that can enhance traditional treatments.

Exploring these therapies requires an open mind and a willingness to integrate different approaches into a comprehensive treatment plan. It's essential to consult with healthcare providers to ensure that any new therapy aligns with individual health needs and does not interfere with existing treatments. By embracing a combination of conventional and alternative therapies, patients can find a balanced approach to managing fibromyalgia and improving their overall quality of life.

ACUPUNCTURE AND MASSAGE

Acupuncture and massage are two of the most widely recognized alternative therapies for managing fibromyalgia symptoms. Both approaches have deep roots in traditional healing practices and have garnered significant attention in modern medicine for their potential benefits in alleviating pain and improving overall well-being.

Acupuncture is an essential part of traditional Chinese medicine. It entails the insertion of very thin needles through the skin at specific locations on the body. According to traditional beliefs, acupuncture works by balancing the flow of energy, or qi, through pathways in the body. In modern scientific terms, acupuncture is thought to stimulate nerves, muscles, and connective tissue, which can boost the body's natural painkillers and increase blood flow. Many fibromyalgia patients report that regular acupuncture sessions help reduce chronic pain and improve sleep quality. It's important to seek treatment from a licensed and experienced acupuncturist to ensure safety and effectiveness.

Massage therapy offers another valuable approach to managing fibromyalgia symptoms. Various types of massage, such as Swedish, deep tissue, and myofascial release, can be particularly beneficial. Massage works by manipulating the body's soft tissues, promoting relaxation, reducing muscle tension, and improving circulation. For fibromyalgia sufferers, massage can help alleviate the widespread muscle pain and stiffness associated with the condition. Regular sessions can also reduce levels of cortisol, the stress hormone, and increase serotonin and dopamine, which can enhance mood and combat depression.

In addition to general massage techniques, specialized forms like *trigger point therapy* and *lymphatic drainage massage* can provide targeted relief. Trigger point therapy focuses on releasing tight muscle knots that cause pain in specific areas, while lymphatic drainage massage helps reduce swelling and improve the lymphatic system's function, which can be beneficial for those experiencing fibromyalgia-related swelling and fluid retention.

Patients exploring these therapies should communicate openly with their therapists about their specific symptoms and sensitivities. Some fibromyalgia sufferers may find certain massage techniques too intense, so it's crucial to start with gentler approaches and adjust based on individual tolerance. Combining acupuncture and massage can provide a comprehensive strategy for managing fibromyalgia, addressing both the physical and emotional dimensions of the condition.

Overall, while acupuncture and massage may not be a cure for fibromyalgia, they offer significant benefits that can complement traditional medical treatments. By incorporating these therapies into a broader treatment plan, patients can achieve better pain management, enhanced relaxation, and improved quality of life. Always consult with your healthcare provider before starting any new therapy to ensure it fits well with your overall treatment plan and health status.

SUPPLEMENTS AND NATURAL REMEDIES

Supplements and natural remedies can significantly aid in managing fibromyalgia symptoms. While not substitutes for medical treatments, they can provide additional relief and support when integrated into a comprehensive treatment plan. Here's a detailed look at some effective options:

Magnesium: This mineral is essential for muscle and nerve function. Many with fibromyalgia find that magnesium supplements help reduce muscle cramps and improve sleep quality. Magnesium citrate and magnesium glycinate are well-absorbed forms. Start with a lower dose to see how your body responds, and consult with your healthcare provider to avoid potential interactions with other medications.

Vitamin D: Adequate vitamin D levels are crucial for bone health and immune function. There's a significant connection between vitamin D deficiency and chronic pain. Ensure your levels are sufficient through a blood test. For those deficient, doctors might recommend a high-dose supplement initially, followed by a maintenance dose. Spending time in sunlight and consuming fatty fish, fortified dairy products, and egg yolks also help maintain healthy levels.

Turmeric/Curcumin: Known for its anti-inflammatory and antioxidant properties, turmeric can help reduce pain and inflammation. Curcumin is the active ingredient and is more effective when taken with black pepper (piperine) to enhance absorption. Supplements often come in doses ranging from 500 to 2,000 mg per day.

Omega-3 Fatty Acids: These essential fats have anti-inflammatory properties that help reduce pain and stiffness. Found in fish oil and flaxseed, they also improve cardiovascular health. Include fatty fish like salmon, mackerel, and sardines in your diet, or take a high-quality fish oil supplement containing EPA and DHA.

Coenzyme Q10 (CoQ10): This antioxidant aids in energy production at the cellular level. Some studies suggest that CoQ10 can reduce fatigue and muscle pain in fibromyalgia patients. Typical doses range from 100 to 200 mg per day.

Melatonin: For those struggling with sleep disturbances, melatonin can be a helpful supplement. It's a hormone that regulates the sleep-wake cycle and can improve sleep quality. Typical doses range from 1 to 3 mg taken about 30 minutes before bedtime. Start with the lowest dose to assess tolerance and effectiveness.

5-HTP (5-Hydroxytryptophan): This supplement is a precursor to serotonin, a neurotransmitter that affects mood and pain perception. It can help with both depression and sleep issues commonly associated with fibromyalgia. Standard doses range from 50 to 100 mg taken before bed. However, it's crucial to use 5-HTP under medical supervision, especially if you're taking other medications for depression or anxiety.

SAM-e (S-adenosylmethionine): This compound, found naturally in the body, helps with mood, pain, and liver health due to its anti-inflammatory and pain-relieving properties. Typical doses range from 200 to 800 mg per day. Start low and increase gradually under a doctor's guidance.

Probiotics: Gut health is often linked to overall health and inflammation. Probiotics can help maintain a healthy gut microbiome, potentially reducing fibromyalgia symptoms. Look for a high-quality probiotic with multiple strains and a high CFU (colony-forming units) count.

Herbal Remedies: Valerian root and CBD oil (cannabidiol) can also be beneficial. Valerian root is a natural sedative that helps with sleep, while CBD oil helps reduce pain and improve sleep quality. Always consult with a healthcare provider before starting any new supplement to ensure safety and appropriateness for your needs.

Integrating these supplements and natural remedies into your treatment plan can help manage fibromyalgia symptoms more effectively. However, it's essential to approach these options with care and always consult with your healthcare provider before starting any new supplement. By combining these natural options with traditional medical treatments, you can achieve a more balanced and effective approach to managing fibromyalgia.

SCIENTIFIC EXPLANATIONS OF ALTERNATIVE THERAPIES

Alternative therapies have long been a topic of interest for those seeking relief from fibromyalgia symptoms. While some approaches lack extensive scientific validation, others have garnered significant research support, illustrating their potential benefits. Understanding the scientific basis of these therapies can help patients make informed decisions about their treatment options.

Acupuncture is a well-known alternative therapy rooted in traditional Chinese medicine. It entails placing fine needles into certain spots on the body to regulate the flow of energy, or "qi." According to recent scientific research, acupuncture can activate the central nervous system, which releases chemicals into the brain, spinal cord, and muscles. The body's innate capacity for healing may be strengthened by these biochemical alterations, which also support mental and physical health. Research has indicated that acupuncture can help reduce pain and improve sleep quality in fibromyalgia patients, making it a valuable complementary therapy.

Massage therapy is another widely recognized alternative treatment. Scientific research suggests that massage can decrease cortisol levels, increase serotonin and dopamine, and reduce muscle tension. These effects collectively contribute to pain relief, relaxation, and improved mood. Studies have shown that regular massage therapy can help alleviate fibromyalgia symptoms, including chronic pain, stiffness, and fatigue. Techniques such as myofascial release, Swedish massage, and deep tissue massage are particularly beneficial for fibromyalgia patients.

Biofeedback is a technique that teaches people how to control physiological processes including heart rate, muscle tension, and blood pressure using visualization and relaxation techniques. Scientific studies have demonstrated that biofeedback can help fibromyalgia patients reduce stress, manage pain, and improve overall quality of life. By learning to regulate their body's responses, patients can gain a greater sense of control over their symptoms.

Tai Chi is a mind-body practice that combines gentle physical movements, meditation, and deep breathing. Research has shown that Tai Chi can significantly improve fibromyalgia symptoms. A study published in the New England Journal of Medicine found that patients who practiced Tai Chi experienced greater improvements in pain, sleep quality, depression, and overall quality of life compared to those who participated in standard stretching exercises. The low-impact nature of Tai Chi makes it an accessible and effective option for individuals with fibromyalgia.

Yoga is another mind-body practice that has gained popularity among fibromyalgia patients. Studies have found that yoga can help reduce pain, improve flexibility, enhance mood, and decrease stress. The practice of yoga involves physical postures, breathing exercises, and meditation, all of which contribute to a holistic approach to managing fibromyalgia symptoms. A 2010 study published in Pain journal found that fibromyalgia patients who participated in a yoga program experienced significant reductions in pain and fatigue compared to those who did not.

Chiropractic care focuses on the diagnosis and treatment of mechanical disorders of the musculoskeletal system, particularly the spine. Some studies suggest that chiropractic adjustments can improve pain and function in fibromyalgia patients by reducing spinal misalignments and improving nervous system function. While more research is needed to fully understand the benefits of chiropractic care for fibromyalgia, many patients report positive outcomes.

Incorporating alternative therapies into a comprehensive fibromyalgia treatment plan can offer significant benefits. While the scientific evidence supporting these therapies varies, many patients find relief through these non-traditional approaches. Consulting with healthcare providers and exploring these options can help individuals with fibromyalgia manage their symptoms more effectively and improve their overall quality of life.

Conclusion

Adding alternative and complementary therapies to your fibromyalgia treatment plan can provide a holistic and personalized approach to managing symptoms. While conventional medications are essential, therapies like acupuncture, massage, Tai Chi, and yoga can enhance your overall well-being by addressing both physical pain and emotional health.

Keep an open dialogue with your healthcare providers to ensure these therapies complement your existing plan. This teamwork can help you find the most effective combination of treatments for managing fibromyalgia.

Incorporating these therapies into your routine empowers you to take an active role in your health, improving symptom control and quality of life. Remember, managing fibromyalgia is an ongoing journey, and exploring various options can help you find the best balance for living well.

CHAPTER 10: PHYSICAL EXERCISE AND MOVEMENT

Physical exercise and movement are crucial elements in managing fibromyalgia. While it may seem counterintuitive to engage in physical activity when dealing with chronic pain, the right types of exercise can significantly reduce symptoms and improve quality of life. This chapter explores the importance of physical activity, specific exercises tailored for fibromyalgia patients, and the benefits of yoga and stretching.

Engaging in regular exercise helps enhance muscle strength, flexibility, and overall stamina. For those with fibromyalgia, exercise is not about pushing to the limits but finding a balance that encourages movement without exacerbating pain. Gentle and low-impact activities, such as walking, swimming, or cycling, are particularly effective. These activities promote cardiovascular health and can be easily adjusted to match individual fitness levels.

Specific exercises tailored to fibromyalgia can address common issues like muscle stiffness, joint pain, and fatigue. These exercises aim to improve mobility and reduce discomfort. The key is to start slow and gradually increase intensity and duration. Consistency is more important than intensity, as regular movement helps maintain benefits over time.

Yoga and stretching offer additional advantages. They combine physical movement with mindfulness, promoting both physical and mental well-being. Yoga's gentle poses and stretching routines can help relieve tension, improve flexibility, and enhance overall relaxation. Incorporating these practices into a daily routine can provide significant relief from fibromyalgia symptoms.

This chapter will provide detailed guidance on how to incorporate these activities into your lifestyle safely and effectively. By understanding the importance of physical activity and adopting a tailored exercise routine, you can take a proactive step toward managing fibromyalgia and improving your overall health.

IMPORTANCE OF PHYSICAL ACTIVITY

Engaging in regular physical activity is vital for managing fibromyalgia symptoms. While it might seem counterintuitive to exercise when experiencing chronic pain and fatigue, physical movement can significantly alleviate these symptoms over time. Exercise helps improve muscle strength, enhances flexibility, and boosts overall stamina, which can make daily activities easier to manage.

One of the primary benefits of physical activity for fibromyalgia patients is its ability to reduce pain. Regular exercise stimulates the release of endorphins, the body's natural painkillers, which can help diminish the perception of pain. Additionally, exercise can improve sleep quality, another crucial aspect of managing fibromyalgia, as poor sleep often exacerbates symptoms.

Moreover, physical activity plays a critical role in combating the stiffness and tension that are common in fibromyalgia. Gentle exercises, such as walking, swimming, or cycling, can help maintain joint mobility and reduce stiffness. These activities also promote better circulation, delivering oxygen and nutrients to muscles and tissues, which can enhance healing and reduce pain.

Mental health benefits are also notable. Physical activity is known to reduce stress, anxiety, and depression, all of which can worsen fibromyalgia symptoms. Exercise provides a sense of accomplishment and boosts self-esteem, contributing to an overall sense of well-being. This holistic approach to managing fibromyalgia acknowledges the interconnectedness of physical and mental health, offering a comprehensive strategy for improvement.

For those new to exercise or experiencing severe symptoms, starting with low-impact activities is crucial. Gradually increasing the intensity and duration of exercise sessions can help prevent overexertion and ensure that physical activity becomes a sustainable part of the daily routine. Consulting with a healthcare provider or a physical therapist can provide personalized guidance tailored to individual capabilities and needs, ensuring that exercise is both safe and effective for managing fibromyalgia.

SPECIFIC EXERCISES FOR FIBROMYALGIA

Selecting the right exercises is crucial for managing fibromyalgia effectively. It's important to choose activities that are low-impact yet effective in enhancing strength, flexibility, and endurance. Here are some specific exercises that are particularly beneficial for individuals with fibromyalgia:

1. **Walking**:
Walking is an excellent low-impact exercise that can be easily adjusted to match one's fitness level. It improves cardiovascular health, boosts mood, and enhances energy levels. Start with short, manageable walks and gradually increase the duration and pace as your stamina improves. Walking outdoors also provides the added benefits of fresh air and a change of scenery, which can be uplifting for mental health.

2. **Swimming and Water Aerobics**:
Exercising in water reduces the strain on joints and muscles, making it an ideal option for fibromyalgia patients. Swimming and water aerobics offer a full-body workout that improves cardiovascular health, strengthens muscles, and enhances flexibility. The buoyancy of water supports the body, reducing pain and stiffness during exercise.

3. **Stretching and Flexibility Exercises**:
Regular stretching helps maintain muscle flexibility and joint range of motion, which can reduce pain and stiffness. Gentle stretches targeting major muscle groups should be incorporated into the daily routine. Holding each stretch for about 30 seconds without bouncing can improve flexibility and prevent muscle tightness.

4. **Strength Training**:

Building muscle strength is essential for supporting joints and improving overall functionality. Using light weights or resistance bands can provide a safe way to perform strength training exercises. Focus on low resistance and high repetitions to avoid overexertion. Exercises like bicep curls, leg lifts, and seated rows can be beneficial.

5. Cycling:

Cycling, whether on a stationary bike or outdoors, is a low-impact activity that can enhance cardiovascular health and build lower body strength. Adjust the bike settings to ensure a comfortable and pain-free experience. Start with short sessions and gradually increase the duration and intensity as your fitness improves.

6. Tai Chi:

Tai Chi is a gentle form of martial arts that involves slow, deliberate movements and deep breathing. It improves balance, flexibility, and muscle strength, while also promoting relaxation and stress reduction. Tai Chi's meditative aspect can help alleviate anxiety and improve overall well-being.

7. Pilates:

Pilates focuses on strengthening the core muscles, improving posture, and enhancing flexibility. It can be particularly beneficial for those with fibromyalgia as it emphasizes controlled movements and breathing. Pilates exercises can be modified to accommodate various fitness levels and physical limitations.

8. Balance Exercises:

Improving balance can prevent falls and enhance overall stability. Simple exercises like standing on one foot, heel-to-toe walking, or using a balance board can be incorporated into your routine. These exercises not only improve physical stability but also enhance body awareness.

9. Low-Impact Aerobics:

Engaging in low-impact aerobic exercises, such as dancing or using an elliptical machine, can increase heart rate and improve cardiovascular fitness without placing excessive stress on the joints. These activities can also be enjoyable and provide a social aspect if done in a group setting.

Incorporating these specific exercises into a regular fitness routine can help manage fibromyalgia symptoms effectively. It's essential to start slowly, listen to your body, and gradually increase the intensity and duration of workouts. Consulting with a physical therapist or a fitness professional who understands fibromyalgia can also provide personalized guidance and ensure that the exercises are both safe and beneficial.

YOGA AND STRETCHING

Yoga and stretching are vital components in managing fibromyalgia symptoms. Both practices offer gentle, low-impact ways to improve flexibility, reduce pain, and enhance overall well-being. Incorporating yoga and regular stretching into your daily routine can significantly alleviate the discomfort associated with fibromyalgia.

Yoga involves a combination of physical postures, breathing exercises, and meditation. It helps in reducing stress, improving flexibility, and strengthening muscles without putting excessive strain on the body. Specific yoga poses, such as Child's Pose, Cat-Cow, and Legs-Up-The-Wall, can be particularly beneficial for those with fibromyalgia. These poses promote relaxation, ease muscle tension, and improve circulation. Additionally, yoga's emphasis on mindful breathing can help manage the anxiety and depression often accompanying fibromyalgia.

One of the key advantages of yoga is its adaptability. Poses can be modified to suit individual capabilities, ensuring that each practice session is safe and effective. Attending a class with an instructor knowledgeable about fibromyalgia can provide personalized guidance and adjustments. For those new to yoga, starting with a gentle or restorative yoga class is advisable to avoid overexertion.

Stretching is equally important for maintaining muscle flexibility and joint mobility. Regular stretching routines can help prevent stiffness and reduce the risk of injury. Focus on gentle, sustained stretches targeting major muscle groups. Hold each stretch for 20-30 seconds, breathing deeply and avoiding any bouncing movements that might cause strain.

A simple yet effective stretching routine might include:

- **Neck Stretches**: Gently tilt your head from side to side and forward and backward to release tension.
- **Shoulder Stretches**: Extend your arm across your chest, holding it with the opposite hand to stretch the shoulder muscles.
- **Hamstring Stretches**: Sit on the floor with one leg extended and the other bent. Reach toward your toes, feeling the stretch along the back of your thigh.
- **Calf Stretches**: Stand facing a wall, step one foot back, and press the heel into the ground to stretch the calf muscles.

Adding yoga and stretching to your daily routine for just 10-15 minutes can significantly help manage fibromyalgia symptoms. Consistency is key, so listen to your body and rest when needed. These gentle practices alleviate physical discomfort and promote inner peace and well-being, creating a holistic approach to managing fibromyalgia.

Conclusion

Incorporating physical exercise and movement into your daily routine is essential for managing fibromyalgia. Regular, low-impact activities like yoga and stretching can improve muscle strength, flexibility, and stamina, reducing pain and discomfort while promoting relaxation and mental well-being. Start slowly and listen to your body, gradually increasing intensity to avoid additional pain. Consistency is crucial for maintaining these benefits over time, enhancing both physical and mental health. Embrace these gentle practices with patience, knowing that each step helps you manage fibromyalgia more effectively.

CHAPTER 11: MENTAL HEALTH AND EMOTIONAL WELL-BEING

Living with fibromyalgia goes beyond managing physical pain and fatigue. The emotional and mental toll of this chronic condition can be equally challenging, if not more so. Anxiety, depression, and stress are common companions of fibromyalgia, often exacerbating physical symptoms and creating a vicious cycle of pain and emotional distress. This chapter delves into the crucial aspect of mental health and emotional well-being for those with fibromyalgia. We will explore various strategies to manage stress, including effective relaxation techniques, the power of mindfulness and meditation, and the invaluable role of psychological support and counseling. Understanding and addressing the emotional components of fibromyalgia can significantly improve quality of life, helping individuals to navigate their daily lives with more resilience and positivity. By integrating these mental health practices, you can create a balanced approach to managing fibromyalgia, one that honors both mind and body.

MANAGING STRESS AND RELAXATION TECHNIQUES FOR FIBROMYALGIA

Effectively managing stress is crucial for individuals with fibromyalgia, as stress can exacerbate symptoms and lead to flare-ups. Implementing stress management and relaxation techniques can help reduce the intensity and frequency of these episodes, enhancing overall well-being.

Deep Breathing Exercises

One effective stress management technique is deep breathing exercises. These exercises can be done anywhere and at any time, providing an immediate sense of calm. By focusing on slow, deep breaths, you can activate your parasympathetic nervous system, which helps lower heart rate and blood pressure, thereby reducing stress levels.

Exercise Example:

- Sit or lie down in a comfortable position.
- Close your eyes and take a deep breath in through your nose, filling your lungs completely.
- Hold your breath for a count of four.
- Exhale slowly through your mouth, emptying your lungs completely.
- Repeat this process for 5-10 minutes, focusing solely on your breathing.

Progressive Muscle Relaxation (PMR)

Progressive muscle relaxation (PMR) is another beneficial technique. PMR involves tensing and then slowly releasing each muscle group in the body, starting from the toes and working up to the head. This method helps identify areas of tension and promotes a state of relaxation throughout the body. Regular practice can lead to significant improvements in muscle relaxation and stress reduction.

Exercise Example:

- Find a quiet place to sit or lie down comfortably.
- Start with your toes, tense the muscles tightly for 5-7 seconds, then release.
- Move up to your calves, thighs, abdomen, chest, arms, and finally your neck and face.
- Focus on the sensation of relaxation after releasing each muscle group.
- Perform this exercise for about 15-20 minutes daily.

Visualization or Guided Imagery

Visualization or guided imagery is a powerful tool for stress management. By imagining peaceful and calming scenes, you can mentally transport yourself to a place of serenity. This practice not only distracts from pain and stress but also engages the mind in a positive and therapeutic way. Listening to guided imagery recordings can enhance this experience and make it more effective.

Exercise Example:

- Sit or lie down in a comfortable position in a quiet space.
- Close your eyes and begin to picture a serene scene, such as a beach, forest, or mountain.
- Focus on the details: the sound of waves, the smell of pine trees, the warmth of the sun.
- Allow yourself to fully immerse in this scene for 10-15 minutes, letting go of any stress or tension.

Regular Physical Activity

Incorporating regular physical activity into your routine is vital. Activities like walking, swimming, or yoga can help release endorphins, the body's natural stress relievers. Exercise doesn't have to be intense; even gentle movement can significantly reduce stress levels and improve mood.

Activity Example:

- Engage in a 30-minute walk daily at a comfortable pace.
- Join a gentle yoga class designed for individuals with chronic pain.
- Swim at a local pool, focusing on gentle strokes that do not strain your muscles.

Creating a Calming Environment

Creating a calming environment is essential for relaxation. Surround yourself with soothing music, calming scents like lavender or chamomile, and soft lighting. Designating a specific area in your home for relaxation activities can provide a retreat from daily stressors.

Setup Example:

- Choose a quiet corner of your home and furnish it with comfortable seating.
- Use a diffuser with calming essential oils like lavender.
- Play soft instrumental music or nature sounds.
- Use warm, dim lighting to create a serene atmosphere.

Establishing a Regular Sleep Routine

Establishing a regular sleep routine is also crucial. Poor sleep can increase stress and worsen fibromyalgia symptoms. Ensure your sleep environment is comfortable, free from electronic devices, and conducive to rest. Practicing good sleep hygiene, like maintaining a consistent sleep schedule and avoiding caffeine before bed, can improve sleep quality and reduce stress.

Routine Example:

- Set a regular wake-up and bedtime for each day.
- Avoid screens (phones, tablets, TVs) for at least an hour before bedtime.
- Create a relaxing pre-sleep routine, such as reading a book or taking a warm bath.

Engaging in Hobbies and Activities You Enjoy

Engaging in hobbies and activities you enjoy is another effective stress management strategy. Whether it's reading, gardening, painting, or any other activity that brings you joy, making time for these pursuits can provide a much-needed break from stress and enhance overall emotional well-being.

Activity Example:

- Dedicate 30 minutes each day to a hobby that relaxes you, such as drawing, knitting, or playing a musical instrument.
- Join a local club or online group related to your hobby to connect with others who share your interests.

Social Support

Social support is also a key factor in managing stress. Connecting with friends, family, or support groups provides an outlet for sharing experiences and receiving encouragement. Knowing that you are not alone in your journey can significantly reduce stress and improve your outlook.

Support Example:

- Schedule regular coffee or phone chats with friends or family.
- Join a local or online support group for individuals with fibromyalgia.
- Participate in community activities or volunteer work to build a network of supportive relationships.

By incorporating these stress management and relaxation techniques into your daily routine, you can better manage fibromyalgia symptoms and improve your quality of life. Regular practice of these methods can lead to long-term benefits, making it easier to cope with the challenges of fibromyalgia.

MINDFULNESS AND MEDITATION

Mindfulness and meditation are powerful tools that can significantly enhance the mental health and emotional well-being of individuals with fibromyalgia. These practices help create a sense of calm, improve focus, and reduce the perception of pain, making them invaluable for managing the daily challenges of this condition.

Mindfulness Exercises

Mindfulness involves paying attention to the present moment without judgment. By focusing on the here and now, you can break free from the cycle of negative thoughts and stress that often accompany chronic pain. Here are some simple mindfulness exercises:

1. **Breathing Exercise***:*

- Sit or lie down in a comfortable position.
- Close your eyes and take a deep breath in through your nose, feeling your abdomen rise.
- Exhale slowly through your mouth, feeling your abdomen fall.
- Focus on your breath and try to maintain a steady rhythm.
- If your mind wanders, gently bring your attention back to your breathing.
- Practice this for 5-10 minutes daily to cultivate a sense of calm.

2. **Observing Your Surroundings***:*

- Choose a quiet place, either indoors or outdoors.
- Sit comfortably and begin to notice your surroundings without labeling them as good or bad.
- Pay attention to the sounds, smells, and sights around you.
- Focus on the details, such as the texture of a leaf or the sound of the wind.
- Spend 5-10 minutes on this exercise, allowing yourself to fully engage with the present moment.

Meditation Techniques

It has been demonstrated that mindfulness meditation, in particular, lowers pain and enhances the quality of life for fibromyalgia sufferers. Here are some meditation techniques to try:

1. Basic Mindfulness Meditation:

- Find a quiet place where you won't be disturbed.
- Sit comfortably with your back straight and hands resting on your lap.
- Shut your eyes and inhale deeply a few times.
- Focus your attention on your breath, feeling the sensation of air entering and leaving your nostrils.
- If your mind wanders, gently bring your attention back to your breath.
- Start with 5 minutes and gradually increase to 20-30 minutes as you become more comfortable.

2. Guided Meditation:

- Use a meditation app or online resource that offers guided meditations.
- Find a comfortable place to sit or lie down.
- Listen to the narrator's voice as they guide you through calming visualizations and breathing techniques.
- Follow along, allowing yourself to be fully immersed in the experience.
- This can be particularly helpful for pain relief and stress reduction.

3. Body Scan Meditation:

- Lie down in a comfortable position with your arms at your sides.
- Shut your eyes and inhale deeply a few times to relax.
- Begin to focus your attention on your toes, noticing any sensations or tension.
- Slowly move your attention up through your body, focusing on each part: feet, legs, hips, abdomen, chest, arms, hands, neck, and head.
- As you focus on each area, imagine releasing any tension and allowing that part of your body to relax.
- Spend 15-20 minutes on this practice, promoting deep relaxation and body awareness.

4. Loving-Kindness Meditation:

- Sit comfortably and close your eyes.
- Take a few deep breaths to center yourself.
- Begin by silently repeating phrases of loving-kindness to yourself: "May I be happy, may I be healthy, may I be safe, may I live with ease."
- After a few minutes, extend these wishes to others, starting with someone you care about, then to acquaintances, and finally to all living beings.

- Spend 10-15 minutes on this practice, fostering a positive mindset and reducing feelings of isolation.

Incorporating Mindfulness and Meditation into Daily Life

Start with just a few minutes each day and gradually increase the time as you become more comfortable. Consistency is key to experiencing the full benefits. You might also consider joining a mindfulness or meditation group, either in person or online, to stay motivated and connect with others who share similar experiences. By embracing mindfulness and meditation, you can develop a more balanced and resilient approach to living with fibromyalgia. These practices offer a way to find peace amidst the pain, enhancing both your mental and emotional well-being. Regular practice can help you cultivate a sense of control and empowerment, making it easier to navigate the ups and downs of life with fibromyalgia.

PSYCHOLOGICAL SUPPORT AND COUNSELING

Psychological support and counseling are crucial components for managing the mental health challenges associated with fibromyalgia. The chronic pain, fatigue, and emotional distress that come with fibromyalgia can significantly impact one's quality of life. Professional counseling can provide the tools and support necessary to cope with these challenges effectively.

Cognitive Behavioral Therapy (CBT) is one of the most effective forms of counseling for individuals with fibromyalgia. CBT focuses on changing negative thought patterns and behaviors that contribute to emotional distress and pain perception. Through CBT, patients learn to identify and challenge harmful thoughts, replacing them with more constructive and positive ones. This can lead to significant improvements in mood, pain management, and overall well-being.

Acceptance and Commitment Therapy (ACT) is another valuable approach. ACT encourages patients to accept their pain and distress as a part of their life, rather than fighting against it. By focusing on their values and committing to actions that align with those values, individuals can improve their mental health and enhance their quality of life. This therapy helps patients develop psychological flexibility, which is crucial for adapting to the ups and downs of living with a chronic condition.

Support groups provide an opportunity for individuals with fibromyalgia to connect with others who understand their experiences. Sharing personal stories, challenges, and successes can foster a sense of community and reduce feelings of isolation. Support groups can be found both in-person and online, offering flexible options for those with varying levels of mobility and comfort.

Individual counseling offers a personalized approach to mental health care. A licensed therapist can work with patients to develop strategies tailored to their specific needs and circumstances. This one-on-one support can be particularly beneficial for addressing issues such as depression, anxiety, and trauma that may be exacerbated by living with fibromyalgia.

Family therapy can also be beneficial, as fibromyalgia not only affects the individual but also their loved ones. Family therapy sessions can help improve communication, understanding, and support within the family unit. This can lead to a more supportive home environment, which is essential for managing the daily challenges of fibromyalgia.

Mindfulness-based stress reduction (MBSR) is another effective therapeutic approach. MBSR combines mindfulness meditation and yoga to help individuals become more aware of their thoughts, feelings, and body sensations. This increased awareness can lead to better stress management and a greater sense of control over one's life.

Finding the right therapist or counselor is an important step in managing fibromyalgia. It is essential to work with a professional who has experience with chronic pain conditions and can offer evidence-based therapies. Patients should feel comfortable and supported by their therapist, ensuring a collaborative and effective therapeutic relationship.

Incorporating psychological support and counseling into a comprehensive fibromyalgia management plan can make a significant difference in mental health and emotional well-being. By addressing the psychological aspects of fibromyalgia, individuals can develop resilience, reduce stress, and improve their overall quality of life. This holistic approach recognizes the interconnectedness of mind and body, promoting healing and well-being on all levels.

Conclusion

Addressing the mental and emotional aspects of fibromyalgia is not just beneficial—it's essential. As we've discussed, effective stress management techniques, regular mindfulness and meditation practices, and seeking psychological support can make a profound difference in your daily life. These strategies empower you to break the cycle of pain and emotional turmoil, fostering a more resilient and positive mindset. By incorporating these practices into your routine, you can cultivate a stronger, more balanced approach to living with fibromyalgia. Remember, it's normal to feel overwhelmed at times, but with the right tools and support, you can navigate these challenges more effectively. Embracing a holistic approach to your well-being, one that includes both physical and mental health, will pave the way for a more fulfilling and manageable life with fibromyalgia. Continue to prioritize your mental health, and don't hesitate to seek out resources and support when needed. Your journey towards better mental and emotional health is a vital component of your overall fibromyalgia management plan.

CHAPTER 12: SLEEP HYGIENE

For many people living with fibromyalgia, insomnia is a frequent and frustrating companion. The chronic pain and discomfort associated with fibromyalgia can make it challenging to achieve restful sleep, leading to a cycle of fatigue and heightened sensitivity to pain. Understanding and implementing effective sleep hygiene practices can significantly improve sleep quality and, in turn, overall well-being.

This chapter delves into practical strategies to enhance your sleep environment and habits, aiming to break the cycle of sleeplessness and pain. From adjusting your bedtime routine to incorporating natural remedies, the goal is to create a sleep-friendly environment that fosters deep, restorative rest. Simple changes, such as maintaining a consistent sleep schedule, reducing screen time before bed, and making dietary adjustments, can make a profound difference.

We will explore a variety of natural remedies, including herbal teas, essential oils, and Epsom salt baths, that can help calm the mind and relax the body. Additionally, we'll discuss the role of melatonin supplements and mindfulness meditation in promoting better sleep. These non-pharmacological approaches offer gentle yet effective ways to enhance sleep quality without the side effects often associated with sleep medications.

By integrating these sleep hygiene practices into your daily routine, you can create a more conducive environment for sleep, ultimately helping to alleviate some of the symptoms of fibromyalgia. Consistent application of these tips and tricks can lead to healthier sleep patterns and a noticeable improvement in your daily life. Let's embark on this journey towards better sleep and improved quality of life together.

IMPROVING SLEEP QUALITY

Sleep is a cornerstone of well-being, particularly for individuals battling fibromyalgia. The pervasive pain and fatigue that accompany this condition can make restorative sleep seem like an unattainable luxury. However, improving sleep quality is not just possible, it is essential for managing symptoms and enhancing overall health. Here's how to create a sleep-friendly environment and establish routines that support better sleep.

Start by prioritizing your sleep environment. Your bedroom should be a sanctuary dedicated to rest. Consider investing in a high-quality mattress and pillows that offer proper support and comfort. The room should be dark, cool, and quiet. Blackout curtains can block disruptive light, while a white noise machine or earplugs can minimize unwanted sounds. If temperature regulation is an issue, breathable, moisture-wicking bed linens can help maintain a comfortable climate.

Establishing a consistent sleep schedule is crucial. Try to go to bed and wake up at the same time every day, even on weekends. This regularity reinforces your body's internal clock, making it easier to fall asleep and wake up naturally. To support this rhythm, expose yourself to natural light during the day and limit exposure to artificial light, especially blue light from screens, in the evening. Consider using blue light filters on devices or switching to activities like reading a physical book before bed.

Developing a pre-sleep routine can signal your body that it's time to wind down. This routine might include calming activities such as taking a warm bath, practicing gentle yoga stretches, or engaging in meditation or deep-breathing exercises. Avoid stimulating activities and heavy meals close to bedtime, as these can interfere with your ability to fall asleep. Caffeine and nicotine are also best avoided in the hours leading up to sleep.

Mindfulness and relaxation techniques are powerful tools for easing into sleep. Progressive muscle relaxation, where you tense and then slowly release each muscle group, can reduce physical tension. Guided imagery or listening to soothing music can also create a peaceful mental state conducive to sleep.

Finally, keep a sleep diary to identify patterns and triggers that affect your sleep. Note what you eat, your activities, and your emotional state, along with details about your sleep quality. This record can reveal habits that need adjustment and serve as a valuable tool when discussing sleep issues with your healthcare provider. Improving sleep quality requires patience and persistence, but the benefits are profound. By creating a supportive sleep environment and establishing healthy routines, you can enhance your rest and, consequently, your overall quality of life with fibromyalgia.

NATURAL REMEDIES AND PRACTICAL TIPS

Finding natural ways to improve sleep can be a game-changer for those with fibromyalgia. Here are some effective, non-pharmacological strategies to help you drift into a restful slumber.

Herbal Teas: Enjoying a calming herbal tea can be a comforting pre-sleep ritual. Chamomile, valerian root, and lavender teas are particularly effective in promoting relaxation and reducing anxiety. For example, a warm cup of chamomile tea before bed can help calm your nerves and prepare your body for sleep. You can also mix these herbs to create a personalized blend that suits your taste and needs.

Essential Oils: Utilize aromatherapy with essential oils like lavender, cedarwood, and bergamot. These oils can be diffused in your room, applied to your pillowcase, or used in a gentle massage to relax your body and mind. For instance, adding a few drops of lavender oil to a diffuser can fill your room with a soothing scent, helping you relax and fall asleep more easily. Alternatively, you can apply diluted lavender oil to your temples and wrists for a direct calming effect.

Epsom Salt Baths: Soaking in a warm bath with Epsom salts can ease muscle tension and pain. The magnesium in Epsom salts can be absorbed through the skin, reducing inflammation and promoting relaxation. Taking a 20-minute bath with Epsom salts before bed can significantly improve your sleep quality. Adding a few drops of lavender oil to the bath can enhance the calming effects.

Melatonin Supplements: Taking melatonin supplements about an hour before bed can help regulate your sleep-wake cycle. Melatonin, a hormone that signals your body to prepare for sleep, can be particularly helpful for those with insomnia. Consult with a healthcare provider to find the right dosage for you, typically starting with a low dose like 0.5 to 1 mg. For example, a small melatonin tablet can help you fall asleep faster and improve your overall sleep quality.

Mindfulness Meditation: Include mindfulness meditation practices such progressive muscle relaxation, guided visualization, and deep breathing. These practices can calm the mind and prepare your body for sleep. Apps like Calm or Headspace offer guided meditations specifically designed to aid sleep. For instance, a 10-minute guided meditation focusing on deep breathing can help reduce stress and promote a peaceful mind before bed.

Dietary Adjustments: Eat foods rich in magnesium, like almonds, spinach, and bananas, to promote relaxation. Avoid heavy, spicy, or acidic foods in the evening to prevent discomfort that might disrupt sleep. For example, a small snack of almonds and a banana an hour before bed can provide the magnesium needed to help your body relax. Additionally, steering clear of caffeine and alcohol in the evening can prevent sleep disturbances.

Routine Adjustments: Establish a consistent bedtime routine. To tell your body it's time to wind down, try reading a book, doing some mild yoga, or listening to soothing music. For instance, setting a specific time each night to start your wind-down routine, such as 9 PM, can help your body and mind transition to sleep mode. Reading a chapter of a book or doing a few gentle yoga stretches can make a significant difference in your sleep quality.

By integrating these natural remedies and practical tips into your daily routine, you can create a conducive environment for better sleep, ultimately enhancing your quality of life. Each small adjustment contributes to a more restful night, helping to manage the symptoms of fibromyalgia more effectively.

Conclusion

Improving sleep hygiene is a powerful tool in managing fibromyalgia symptoms. By focusing on natural remedies and practical tips, you can create a bedtime routine that promotes relaxation and restorative sleep. The strategies discussed in this chapter are designed to help you fall asleep more easily and enjoy a deeper, more refreshing sleep.

Remember, small changes can have a big impact. Incorporating practices such as drinking calming herbal teas, using essential oils for aromatherapy, taking Epsom salt baths, and practicing mindfulness meditation can significantly improve your sleep quality. Additionally, making dietary adjustments and maintaining a consistent bedtime routine can help set the stage for a restful night.

It's essential to remain patient and consistent as you implement these changes. Adapting new habits takes time, but the benefits are well worth the effort. Improved sleep can lead to reduced pain, better mood, and increased energy levels, all of which contribute to a better quality of life for those living with fibromyalgia.

CONCLUSION TO PART III: TREATMENTS AND SYMPTOM MANAGEMENT

As we conclude Part III, it's essential to recognize that managing fibromyalgia is a multifaceted journey that requires a combination of medical, lifestyle, and holistic approaches. The treatments and symptom management strategies discussed throughout this section are designed to provide a broad spectrum of options, allowing for a personalized and adaptable approach to care.

First and foremost, the medical and pharmacological treatments offer critical relief from the primary symptoms of fibromyalgia. By understanding the various medications available, including their benefits and potential side effects, patients can work collaboratively with their healthcare providers to develop an effective treatment plan. This tailored approach ensures that the chosen medications align with individual health profiles and symptom patterns, optimizing outcomes.

Complementary and alternative therapies also play a significant role in managing fibromyalgia. Therapies such as acupuncture, massage, and the use of supplements offer additional layers of relief and support. These therapies, often rooted in ancient practices and now supported by modern scientific research, provide valuable tools for addressing pain, reducing inflammation, and promoting relaxation. The exploration of these therapies highlights their potential to enhance conventional treatment plans, offering patients a more holistic and comprehensive approach to care.

Physical exercise and movement are indispensable in the management of fibromyalgia. Engaging in regular, targeted exercise helps to alleviate pain, increase mobility, and boost overall energy levels. The specific exercises and routines provided in this section are designed to be gentle yet effective, accommodating varying levels of physical capability. By incorporating these exercises into daily life, patients can experience significant improvements in their physical and mental well-being.

Mental health and emotional resilience are equally critical. Techniques such as stress management, mindfulness, and meditation provide powerful tools for coping with the emotional challenges of fibromyalgia. By fostering a positive mindset and reducing stress, patients can improve their overall quality of life. This section underscores the importance of mental health as a fundamental component of comprehensive fibromyalgia management.

Lastly, improving sleep hygiene is a cornerstone of effective symptom management. Quality sleep is crucial for healing and daily functioning, yet many with fibromyalgia struggle with sleep disturbances. The tips and natural remedies provided here offer practical solutions for achieving better sleep, helping to break the cycle of pain and fatigue.

In summary, the treatments and strategies discussed in Part III provide a robust framework for managing fibromyalgia. By integrating medical treatments with complementary therapies, physical exercise, mental health practices, and sleep hygiene, patients can develop a well-rounded and effective approach to care. This holistic strategy not only addresses the multifaceted nature of fibromyalgia but also empowers patients to take control of their health and well-being. The journey to managing fibromyalgia is unique for each individual, but with the right tools and knowledge, a better quality of life is within reach.

PART 4: LIVING WITH FIBROMYALGIA

Living with fibromyalgia often feels like navigating an uncharted territory, filled with constant pain, fatigue, and a myriad of other symptoms that disrupt daily life. The journey to a diagnosis can be long and fraught with frustration, as patients often encounter disbelief and misdiagnoses. Yet, within this challenging landscape, there are remarkable stories of resilience, hope, and triumph. These stories are not just anecdotes but powerful testaments to the human spirit's capacity to endure and overcome adversity.

In this chapter, we delve into the personal narratives of individuals who have faced the trials of fibromyalgia head-on. These stories highlight their struggles, the winding paths to their diagnoses, and the strategies they employed to reclaim their lives. Through their experiences, we gain invaluable insights into the diverse ways people manage this condition, offering a beacon of hope and a wealth of practical advice for others on similar journeys.

For instance, we meet Grace, an artist who transformed her creative process to accommodate her new reality and found strength in community support. Ethan, a single father, turned his personal battle into advocacy, helping others understand and cope with fibromyalgia. Mia, a dynamic marketing executive, adapted her professional life to her needs and emerged as a mentor for those newly diagnosed. Each story is unique, yet they all share a common thread of resilience and adaptability.

These narratives are more than mere testimonials; they are blueprints of hope. They demonstrate that, despite the unpredictable and often debilitating nature of fibromyalgia, there are ways to lead fulfilling lives. By sharing their journeys, these individuals provide not only encouragement but also concrete strategies that readers can apply in their own lives. Their stories remind us that while fibromyalgia may shape our experiences, it does not define our potential for joy and accomplishment.

CHAPTER 13: PATIENT STORIES

INSIGHTS FROM OUR FIBROMYALGIA COMMUNITY: A SURVEY ON LIVING WITH CHRONIC PAIN

Living with fibromyalgia is a journey filled with challenges that can be difficult to understand unless experienced firsthand. To gain a deeper insight into the daily struggles and triumphs of those affected, I personally conducted a survey targeting individuals living with fibromyalgia. The goal was to gather firsthand accounts and data that could illuminate the realities of this condition, helping others feel seen and understood. The responses we received provide a poignant glimpse into the lives of our fibromyalgia community.

Demographics and Duration of Diagnosis

Our survey reached a diverse group of individuals spanning various age groups, from mid-30s to 65 and older. This diversity offers a broad perspective on how fibromyalgia impacts individuals at different stages of life. Many respondents have been living with fibromyalgia for over a decade, emphasizing the chronic nature of this condition and the long-term challenges they face.

Common Symptoms

Respondents shared a range of symptoms, with widespread pain, fatigue, and sleep disturbances being the most commonly reported. Additionally, many individuals experience cognitive difficulties, often referred to as "fibro fog," along with headaches and gastrointestinal issues such as irritable bowel syndrome. These symptoms collectively highlight the multifaceted and often overwhelming nature of fibromyalgia.

Pain Severity

Pain severity varied among respondents, with some experiencing mild to moderate pain and others enduring severe, debilitating pain. This variability underscores the unique and personal nature of each individual's experience with fibromyalgia, reinforcing that there is no one-size-fits-all approach to managing this condition.

Effective Treatments

Individuals in the study reported various effective strategies for symptom control. Many found benefits from doctor-prescribed drugs, regular physical activity, and nutritional supplements. Physiotherapy sessions and common pain medications available without prescription were also cited as helpful. Some participants experienced improvement through complementary treatments like acupuncture and therapeutic massage. These diverse approaches highlight the importance of tailoring treatment plans to each person's unique needs, often combining multiple methods for optimal results.

Messages from the Fibromyalgia Community

A powerful theme emerged from the survey responses: the need for greater understanding and patience from others. Many participants expressed the desire for recognition that fibromyalgia is a legitimate and debilitating condition, not a result of laziness or emotional weakness. They emphasized the importance of empathy and support from family, friends, and the broader community.

Respondents also highlighted the significant impact of fibromyalgia on daily life. The fluctuating nature of the condition, with symptom severity varying greatly from day to day, makes maintaining a consistent routine challenging. This unpredictability adds an extra layer of difficulty to managing their lives.

Conclusion

The insights from our survey provide a comprehensive and empathetic look at the experiences of those living with fibromyalgia. By sharing these findings, we hope to foster a deeper understanding and create a more supportive community. Recognizing the individual challenges and needs of those with fibromyalgia is crucial in helping them lead better, more manageable lives.

STORIES OF HOPE AND RESILIENCE

EMMA'S JOURNEY: FINDING STRENGTH IN ADVERSITY

At 38, Emma was a successful advertising professional thriving in the bustling atmosphere of Chicago. Her career was fulfilling, and she relished the city's dynamic environment and her lively social circle. However, her life took an unexpected turn when she began experiencing unexplained discomfort and exhaustion. Following a series of medical consultations and examinations spanning several months, Emma received a diagnosis of fibromyalgia. This news left her devastated, feeling as though her once-vibrant lifestyle was now out of reach.

The initial shock of the diagnosis deeply affected Emma. She found it challenging to maintain her work performance and felt disconnected from friends who struggled to grasp the nature of her condition. Emma's perspective shifted when she became part of a community support network for individuals with fibromyalgia. Interacting with others who shared their experiences and management strategies rekindled her optimism.

Determined to adapt, Emma made substantial changes to her lifestyle. She transitioned to a role that offered remote work options and allowed her to tailor her schedule to her fluctuating energy levels. She incorporated gentle stretching exercises and mindfulness practices into her routine, while also adopting a nutritious diet focused on reducing inflammation. Gradually, Emma began to regain a sense of control over her daily life. Although her symptoms persisted, she developed effective coping mechanisms. Now, Emma dedicates her time to raising awareness about fibromyalgia and inspiring others facing similar challenges to find their inner strength.

DAVID'S BATTLE: EMBRACING A NEW NORMAL

David, a 45-year-old father of two, had always been the family's pillar of strength. He worked as a construction manager, a physically demanding job that he loved. When David began experiencing severe pain and exhaustion, he brushed it off as part of the job. However, the symptoms worsened, leading to his fibromyalgia diagnosis.

The diagnosis was a tough pill to swallow for David. His job became increasingly difficult, and he worried about supporting his family. David's wife, Sarah, became his rock, helping him navigate this new reality. She researched extensively about fibromyalgia and found ways to adjust their family life to support David's health. They implemented a strict bedtime routine to improve his sleep and focused on nutrient-rich meals that alleviated some of his symptoms.

David also found solace in a local fibromyalgia community. He met others who faced similar struggles and shared their stories of resilience. Inspired, David started a blog to document his experiences and connect with others battling the condition. Through writing and community support, David found a new purpose. He learned to pace himself, accepting that it was okay to ask for help and take breaks. Though he could no longer work as he once did, David's spirit of resilience never waned. He now champions for better understanding and support for fibromyalgia patients.

SOPHIA'S RESILIENCE: REDISCOVERING JOY IN LIFE

Sophia was a 52-year-old artist whose life revolved around creativity. Her paintings were her passion and her livelihood. When fibromyalgia struck, the constant pain in her hands and fatigue made it nearly impossible to continue her work. For Sophia, the loss was deeply personal, shaking her identity to its core.

Depression set in, and Sophia withdrew from friends and family. Her breakthrough came during an art therapy session recommended by her therapist. She found that expressing her pain through art was cathartic. Sophia began to explore different mediums that were less strenuous on her hands, such as digital art and photography.

Through these new forms of expression, Sophia rediscovered her joy. She started an online gallery to showcase her work and connect with other artists facing similar challenges. This venture not only revived her passion but also provided her with a supportive community. Sophia's art now focuses on themes of resilience and healing, inspiring others to find beauty and strength in adversity.

These stories highlight the profound resilience of individuals living with fibromyalgia. Through community support, lifestyle changes, and newfound passions, they have transformed their lives, offering hope and inspiration to others on similar journeys.

SARAH'S TRIUMPH: REDISCOVERING STRENGTH AND PURPOSE

Sarah was a 34-year-old teacher who loved inspiring her students. When she started experiencing constant pain and fatigue, she thought it was due to the stress of her demanding job. Multiple visits to doctors led to various misdiagnoses, from chronic fatigue syndrome to depression. It took almost two years for her to finally be diagnosed with fibromyalgia. The journey was emotionally and physically exhausting, filled with frustration and hopelessness.

After the diagnosis, Sarah felt a sense of relief but also a new set of challenges. She struggled to find effective treatments and balance her teaching career with her health needs. Her breakthrough came when she met a rheumatologist who specialized in fibromyalgia. Together, they developed a comprehensive treatment plan that included medication, physical therapy, and a structured exercise regime focusing on low-impact activities like swimming and yoga.

Sarah also discovered the power of mindfulness and meditation, which helped her manage her pain and reduce stress. She joined a support group for fibromyalgia patients and found comfort in sharing her experiences with others who truly understood her struggles. Over time, Sarah regained control over her life. She adjusted her work schedule to part-time, allowing her to rest and manage her symptoms more effectively. Today, she uses her experience to educate her students and colleagues about fibromyalgia, fostering a supportive and understanding environment.

JAMES' ODYSSEY: OVERCOMING MISUNDERSTANDING AND PAIN

James, a 42-year-old software engineer, had always been in good health. When he began to experience severe muscle pain and debilitating fatigue, he was perplexed. His journey to a fibromyalgia diagnosis was fraught with skepticism from medical professionals who attributed his symptoms to stress and anxiety. It took three years of relentless persistence and multiple doctor visits to finally receive the correct diagnosis.

James felt a mix of relief and despair upon his diagnosis. He faced the challenge of finding effective treatments while managing his demanding job. With the support of his wife, he explored various treatment options, from medications to alternative therapies like acupuncture and massage. It was through a combination of these treatments that he found significant relief.

James also accepted a change in lifestyle, embracing regular exercise and a well-balanced diet full of foods high in anti-inflammatory properties. He found solace in practicing Tai Chi, which helped improve his flexibility and reduce pain. By making these changes, James not only managed his symptoms but also improved his overall well-being.

Today, James is an advocate for fibromyalgia awareness in the tech industry. He has started a blog to share his journey and tips for managing the condition, providing support and hope to others in similar situations.

Lisa was a 29-year-old mother of two when she began experiencing widespread pain and chronic fatigue. Her journey to a diagnosis was particularly challenging due to her young age and the dismissal of her symptoms by multiple healthcare providers. For over four years, Lisa was misdiagnosed with conditions ranging from rheumatoid arthritis to anxiety disorders. The eventual diagnosis of fibromyalgia came as both a relief and a daunting new reality.

Determined to find a way to live well with fibromyalgia, Lisa delved into extensive research and tried various treatments. She found that a combination of physical therapy, gentle stretching exercises, and a strict sleep schedule significantly improved her symptoms. Lisa also discovered the benefits of a plant-based diet, which helped reduce inflammation and boost her energy levels.

Support from her family played a crucial role in Lisa's journey. Her husband took on more responsibilities at home, allowing her to focus on her health. She also connected with other fibromyalgia patients through online forums, where she found invaluable advice and emotional support.

Lisa's resilience paid off. She now manages her symptoms effectively and has even started a local support group for young mothers with fibromyalgia. By sharing her story and strategies, Lisa inspires others to persevere and find their path to a fulfilling life despite the challenges of fibromyalgia.

These stories of Sarah, James, and Lisa highlight the resilience and strength required to navigate life with fibromyalgia. Their journeys of misdiagnosis, struggle, and eventual triumph offer hope and inspiration to others facing similar challenges.

TESTIMONIALS AND COPING STRATEGIES

GRACE'S JOURNEY: EMBRACING ADAPTATION AND STRENGTH

Grace, a 37-year-old artist, lived a vibrant life filled with creativity and passion. When she began experiencing persistent pain and fatigue, her world was turned upside down. The road to her fibromyalgia diagnosis was long and frustrating, filled with countless doctor visits and misdiagnoses. Initially labeled as suffering from stress and overwork, it took nearly four years for her to receive the correct diagnosis.

Receiving the diagnosis was a bittersweet moment for Grace. She was relieved to finally have an explanation for her suffering but also daunted by the chronic nature of the condition. Determined to reclaim her life, Grace immersed herself in understanding fibromyalgia. She realized that while she couldn't cure her condition, she could learn to manage it effectively.

Grace found solace in routine and structure. She began incorporating gentle yoga and tai chi into her daily routine, which helped alleviate some of her pain and improved her flexibility. Meditation and deep-breathing exercises became essential tools in managing her stress and anxiety. By focusing on her mental health, she found a significant reduction in her physical symptoms.

A major factor in Grace's fibromyalgia management was dietary adjustments. Her pain levels decreased when she switched to an anti-inflammatory diet full of fruits, vegetables, and omega-3 fatty acids. Grace also found that eliminating processed foods and sugars made a noticeable difference in her energy levels.

The support from her family and friends was invaluable. Grace's husband became her biggest advocate, helping her navigate the complexities of the medical system and ensuring she had the support she needed. Her close-knit circle of friends provided emotional support, understanding when she had to cancel plans or needed extra help.

Art remained a therapeutic outlet for Grace. She adapted her creative process to accommodate her new limitations, finding new ways to express herself without exacerbating her symptoms. Grace started teaching art classes, sharing her passion and coping strategies with others who had similar conditions. Her classes became a community of support and encouragement, a testament to her resilience and adaptability.

ETHAN'S TALE: FROM ISOLATION TO ADVOCACY

Ethan, a 45-year-old single father, faced significant challenges when he started experiencing severe pain and exhaustion. His path to diagnosis was riddled with disbelief from doctors who attributed his symptoms to psychological issues. It took nearly five years before a compassionate rheumatologist diagnosed him with fibromyalgia.

Ethan's initial reaction was a mix of relief and despair. Understanding his condition allowed him to stop questioning his sanity, but the chronic nature of fibromyalgia was overwhelming. As a single father, he worried about his ability to care for his children and maintain his job.

Determined to find a way forward, Ethan explored various treatment options. He found that a combination of medication, physical therapy, and acupuncture significantly improved his quality of life. Regular sessions with a physical therapist helped him develop an exercise routine that increased his strength and stamina without triggering flare-ups.

Support networks became a lifeline for Ethan. He joined an online support group for men with fibromyalgia, finding solidarity and understanding that he struggled to find elsewhere. These connections provided practical advice and emotional support, helping him navigate the complexities of living with chronic pain.

Ethan also discovered the importance of pacing himself. He learned to listen to his body, resting when necessary and breaking tasks into manageable steps. This approach reduced the frequency of his flare-ups and allowed him to maintain a semblance of normalcy in his daily life.

Inspired by his journey, Ethan became an advocate for fibromyalgia awareness. He started a blog to share his experiences, offering tips and encouragement to others struggling with the condition. His advocacy work extended to speaking at local events and collaborating with healthcare providers to improve understanding and support for fibromyalgia patients.

MIA'S RESILIENCE: TRANSFORMING STRUGGLE INTO EMPOWERMENT

Mia, a 32-year-old marketing executive, was always on the go. When she began to experience debilitating pain and chronic fatigue, her active lifestyle came to a halt. The path to her fibromyalgia diagnosis was long and filled with skepticism from medical professionals who dismissed her symptoms as stress-related. It took nearly three years and countless consultations before she was correctly diagnosed. Upon diagnosis, Mia felt a mix of relief and fear. While she finally had a name for her suffering, the realization that it was a chronic condition was daunting. Determined not to let fibromyalgia define her, Mia took proactive steps to manage her condition.

Mia found that a multidisciplinary approach worked best for her. She incorporated medication, physical therapy, and cognitive-behavioral therapy into her routine. Regular sessions with a physiotherapist helped her maintain mobility and reduce pain, while cognitive-behavioral therapy provided her with tools to manage the mental toll of living with chronic illness.

Dietary changes also played a significant role in Mia's management strategy. She adopted a gluten-free, anti-inflammatory diet, which helped reduce her pain and improve her energy levels. Hydration and regular, balanced meals became essential components of her daily routine.

Support from her workplace was crucial in Mia's journey. She worked with her employer to create a flexible work schedule that accommodated her needs. This flexibility allowed her to rest when necessary and maintain her productivity without exacerbating her symptoms.

Mia also discovered the power of community. She joined a local fibromyalgia support group where she found understanding and camaraderie. Sharing her experiences and learning from others provided emotional relief and practical tips for managing her condition.

Empowered by her journey, Mia became a mentor for others with fibromyalgia. She started an online support group and regularly hosted webinars to share her coping strategies and offer support. Her story of resilience and empowerment inspired many, proving that life with fibromyalgia, while challenging, could still be fulfilling and purposeful.

Conclusion

The stories shared in this chapter serve as powerful reminders that living with fibromyalgia, while undeniably challenging, is also a journey marked by resilience, adaptability, and hope. Each narrative underscores the importance of finding personal strategies that work, whether through medical treatment, lifestyle adjustments, or community support. These accounts are not just testimonials but lifelines for others navigating similar paths.

In reading about Grace, Ethan, and Mia, we see the diverse ways individuals can reclaim their lives from fibromyalgia. Their experiences offer practical advice and emotional support, showing that it is possible to find balance and fulfillment despite the condition. These stories encourage us to seek out what works best for us and to remain hopeful, knowing that we are not alone in our struggles.

CHAPTER 14: COMMUNITY SUPPORT

Navigating life with fibromyalgia can be daunting and isolating. However, building a solid community support system can significantly alleviate the daily struggles associated with this condition. **Community support encompasses both online resources and in-person networks** that provide emotional solace, practical advice, and a sense of belonging. For many living with fibromyalgia, finding people who understand their pain can be a lifeline. It's not just about sympathy; it's about genuine empathy from those who walk the same path.

The advent of the internet has revolutionized how support is accessed. **Online resources and support groups** have emerged as invaluable tools for those seeking connection and advice. These digital platforms provide a space for sharing experiences, offering tips, and simply venting frustrations. They can be accessed anytime, offering 24/7 support that is particularly comforting during sleepless nights or flare-ups.

But online interactions, while incredibly beneficial, are just one part of the support spectrum. **Building a tangible support network within your local community** can be equally, if not more, impactful. This network might include family, friends, healthcare providers, and even local community groups. Each element of this network plays a unique role in providing comprehensive support that addresses both the physical and emotional challenges of fibromyalgia.

Understanding how to harness these resources and cultivate a support system is crucial. This chapter will delve into various ways to connect with others, both online and offline, to create a robust network of support. Whether through a local fibromyalgia support group, an online forum, or regular visits with a therapist, the goal is to surround yourself with a community that understands, supports, and uplifts you.

ONLINE RESOURCES AND SUPPORT GROUPS

Navigating the complexities of fibromyalgia can feel overwhelming, but connecting with others who share similar experiences can provide much-needed support and understanding. Online resources and support groups offer invaluable opportunities for individuals to share their stories, learn from others, and find solace in knowing they are not alone.

Online forums Many websites host communities where people with fibromyalgia can discuss symptoms, treatments, and coping strategies. These forums are rich with shared experiences, offering insights that might not be available in medical literature. Participating in these discussions can help you feel connected and informed.

Social media platforms also host numerous fibromyalgia support groups. These groups allow members to post updates, ask questions, and share resources. They are often moderated to ensure a safe and supportive environment. Engaging with these communities can provide real-time advice and emotional support.

Specialized websites dedicated to fibromyalgia offer comprehensive resources, including the latest research, treatment options, and personal stories. They often have sections dedicated to patient education, providing in-depth information about managing fibromyalgia. These websites can be a reliable source of information and updates about the condition.

Virtual support groups have gained popularity, especially with the rise of telehealth. Various organizations offer online meetings where you can interact with others through video calls. These virtual meetings can be particularly beneficial if you prefer a more personal interaction or if local in-person groups are not available in your area.

Mobile apps designed for chronic illness management, provide platforms for tracking symptoms, medications, and sharing progress with a community of users. These apps often include forums and chat features, allowing for instant connection and support.

Webinars and online workshops are also excellent resources. Many organizations host educational sessions covering various aspects of fibromyalgia, from pain management to mental health. These events often feature experts in the field and offer a chance to ask questions and engage in discussions. Participating in these webinars can enhance your knowledge and provide practical tips for daily living.

In addition to these online resources, **local support groups** often have an online presence where you can find information about meetings and events. Various platforms can help you find local groups dedicated to fibromyalgia support. Attending these groups, whether virtually or in-person, can foster a sense of community and provide ongoing support.

By leveraging these online resources and support groups, you can build a robust support network that provides not only information and advice but also emotional and social connections. This network can play a crucial role in managing fibromyalgia, helping you feel empowered and less isolated. Engaging with others who understand your journey can be incredibly uplifting and can provide the encouragement needed to navigate the challenges of fibromyalgia.

BUILDING A SUPPORT NETWORK

Creating a robust support network is crucial for those living with fibromyalgia. While dealing with the daily challenges of this condition, having a reliable circle of support can make a significant difference. It provides emotional strength, practical help, and a sense of belonging.

Start by **identifying the people in your life** who are understanding and empathetic. These could be family members, close friends, or even colleagues who have shown compassion towards your condition. Having open and honest conversations with them about your struggles and needs can pave the way for their support. Explain what fibromyalgia is, how it affects you, and the kind of assistance you might require. Education is key, as it helps them understand your condition better and how best to help you.

Joining local **support groups** can also be incredibly beneficial. These groups provide a space where you can share experiences, learn from others, and find solace in knowing you are not alone. Meeting others who understand what you're going through can be incredibly comforting. These interactions can provide practical advice on managing symptoms and navigating daily life. Additionally, these groups often organize activities and workshops that can offer new insights and coping strategies.

Don't underestimate the power of **professional support**. Therapists and counselors can provide invaluable guidance. Cognitive-behavioral therapy, for instance, can help you develop strategies to manage pain and stress. A therapist can also assist in improving your mental health, which is closely tied to physical well-being. Sometimes, the burden of fibromyalgia can lead to feelings of isolation or depression, and professional help can provide the tools to handle these emotions effectively.

Neighbors and community organizations can also be part of your support network. Sometimes, neighbors can assist with daily tasks that might be challenging for you, like running errands or providing a ride to medical appointments. Community organizations often have volunteer programs designed to help those in need, which can be a great resource.

Building an online network can complement your local support system. Social media groups and online forums offer a platform to connect with others worldwide who share your condition. These online communities can provide advice, share resources, and offer a space to vent and be heard. They can be particularly useful for those times when you need support outside of regular group meeting hours.

Maintaining and nurturing these relationships is essential. Regularly updating your support network about your condition and needs can help them provide better support. Showing appreciation for their help also strengthens these bonds. Small gestures of gratitude can go a long way in maintaining a supportive relationship.

Finally, consider creating a **personal care team**. This could include your primary care physician, specialists, a physical therapist, and a nutritionist. Regularly communicating with your care team about your symptoms and treatment progress can help them tailor their advice and care to your specific needs. A well-coordinated care team can ensure that all aspects of your health are being addressed, providing a more comprehensive support system.

In summary, building a support network involves reaching out to those around you, joining local and online groups, seeking professional help, and maintaining these relationships with regular communication and appreciation. This network can provide the emotional, practical, and medical support needed to manage fibromyalgia effectively, helping you to lead a more fulfilling and balanced life.

Conclusion

In the journey of managing fibromyalgia, **community support stands as a pillar of strength**. By actively seeking and nurturing both online and offline support networks, individuals can find the empathy and practical help they need. These connections not only provide emotional relief but also offer practical strategies to manage daily challenges. The shared experiences within these communities foster a sense of belonging and understanding, which is essential for mental and emotional well-being. Remember, you are not alone—reaching out and connecting with others can transform your experience and provide the support needed to navigate life with fibromyalgia.

CHAPTER 15: DAILY MANAGEMENT STRATEGIES

Living with fibromyalgia presents unique challenges that require a well-structured approach to daily life. The unpredictability of symptoms like pain, fatigue, and cognitive fog makes it essential to develop effective management strategies. This chapter aims to provide practical and actionable advice to help individuals navigate their daily routines more efficiently and with less strain. By focusing on planning and organization, adapting daily life, and mastering time and energy management techniques, we can create a framework that enhances quality of life despite the limitations imposed by fibromyalgia.

One of the most critical aspects of managing fibromyalgia is the ability to plan and organize effectively. Proper planning helps prioritize tasks, reduce unnecessary stress, and ensure that energy is conserved for the most important activities. For instance, creating a daily schedule that balances activities and rest periods can prevent overexertion and reduce the likelihood of flare-ups. Tools like planners, to-do lists, and digital apps can assist in keeping track of tasks and appointments, making it easier to manage time and responsibilities.

Adapting daily life to accommodate fibromyalgia involves making modifications that reduce physical strain and enhance comfort. Simple changes, such as using ergonomic tools in the kitchen or adjusting the height of a work desk, can make a significant difference. It's also important to create a living environment that supports relaxation and reduces stress. This might include incorporating soothing colors in home decor, using aromatherapy, or setting up a dedicated space for rest and meditation.

Time and energy management techniques are crucial for maintaining productivity while managing fibromyalgia. These strategies focus on balancing activity with rest, setting realistic goals, and recognizing personal limits. Techniques like pacing, where activities are broken down into manageable chunks with frequent breaks, can help conserve energy and prevent burnout. Delegating tasks and asking for help when needed are also essential components of effective energy management. People dealing with fibromyalgia can enhance their quality of life by adopting everyday coping techniques. The goal is to create a personalized schedule that allows for accomplishing tasks while also prioritizing adequate relaxation. By fine-tuning these practices, those affected by fibromyalgia can navigate their day-to-day activities more effectively, leading to a sense of empowerment and improved health outcomes. Striking the right balance between staying active and getting enough rest is crucial for maintaining a rewarding lifestyle, even in the face of fibromyalgia's obstacles.

PLANNING AND ORGANIZATION

Living with fibromyalgia requires a strategic approach to daily management, focusing on planning and organization. Establishing a structured routine can significantly reduce stress and help manage symptoms more effectively. **Creating a daily schedule that prioritizes tasks and allocates time for rest** is essential. For instance, breaking the day into manageable segments with specific time slots for activities and rest periods can prevent overexertion and help maintain energy levels throughout the day.

Start by identifying the most critical tasks that need to be accomplished and arrange them according to your energy levels. Morning hours might be more productive for some, while others may find the afternoon more suitable for demanding tasks. Use a planner or digital calendar to keep track of appointments, medications, and other important activities. This not only helps in staying organized but also ensures that nothing important is overlooked.

To further streamline daily activities, consider **meal planning and preparation**. This involves deciding on meals for the week ahead and preparing ingredients or entire meals in advance. Not only does this save time and energy on busy days, but it also ensures you maintain a healthy diet that supports your well-being. For example, preparing a batch of healthy snacks or cooking double portions and freezing half can be a game-changer on days when cooking feels overwhelming.

Incorporating assistive tools and technologies can also enhance your organizational efforts. **Voice-activated assistants, reminder apps, and automated services** can handle routine tasks, allowing you to conserve energy for more essential activities. For instance, setting up reminders for medication or using grocery delivery services can reduce the physical and mental burden of these tasks. Moreover, delegating tasks to family members or friends when possible can make a significant difference. **Communicating openly about your limitations and asking for help** with specific chores or responsibilities can lighten your load. This might include asking a family member to handle grocery shopping or requesting assistance with household chores. Remember, accepting help is not a sign of weakness but a strategic way to manage your condition more effectively.

Another crucial aspect of planning and organization is creating a **flexible mindset**. Fibromyalgia symptoms can be unpredictable, and having the ability to adjust your plans without guilt or frustration is vital. If a flare-up occurs, allow yourself to reschedule or delegate tasks. Maintaining flexibility in your approach ensures that you can adapt to changing circumstances without compromising your well-being.

To illustrate, consider Jane, a fibromyalgia patient who found relief in meticulously planning her week. She used color-coded calendars to differentiate between high-energy and low-energy tasks. By incorporating regular rest breaks and allowing flexibility for flare-ups, Jane managed to maintain a balanced lifestyle that accommodated her condition. Her planning also included setting up a support system where family members pitched in during tough times, ensuring she wasn't overwhelmed.

In essence, effective planning and organization are about creating a supportive structure that accommodates the ebb and flow of fibromyalgia. By prioritizing tasks, utilizing technology, and embracing flexibility, you can navigate daily life more smoothly, ensuring you conserve energy for the things that matter most.

ADAPTING DAILY LIFE

Adapting daily life with fibromyalgia involves finding ways to make everyday tasks manageable and less draining. One of the most effective strategies is simplifying routines to conserve energy. This can be achieved by **modifying your environment** and using adaptive tools. For example, in the kitchen, consider using electric can openers, lightweight cookware, and ergonomic utensils to minimize strain and effort. Setting up a workstation that reduces the need for repetitive movements can also help, such as keeping frequently used items within easy reach to avoid unnecessary bending or stretching.

Another essential aspect of adapting daily life is **prioritizing tasks** based on their importance and urgency. Developing a habit of assessing your to-do list and focusing on what truly needs to be done can help manage your energy better. For instance, on days when symptoms are more intense, it might be wise to postpone less critical activities and focus on essential tasks only. This prioritization can also extend to social commitments, ensuring you reserve your energy for interactions that are most meaningful or necessary.

Pacing yourself is another crucial technique. This means breaking activities into smaller, more manageable chunks and spreading them throughout the day or week. If cleaning the house is overwhelming, try tackling one room at a time with breaks in between. Similarly, for work-related tasks, take short, frequent breaks to avoid overexertion and prevent symptom flare-ups. This approach not only helps in maintaining productivity but also reduces the risk of exacerbating pain and fatigue.

Incorporating **assistive devices and technology** can significantly enhance daily functioning. Tools like grab bars in the bathroom, raised toilet seats, and shower chairs can make personal care tasks safer and less tiring. For mobility, consider using aids such as walking sticks or mobility scooters if needed. Technology can also play a role, from smart home devices that automate daily tasks to apps that help track symptoms and manage medications.

For example, Sarah, a fibromyalgia patient, found immense relief in reorganizing her home to reduce physical exertion. She installed pull-out shelves in her kitchen to avoid bending and reaching, and she used a voice-activated assistant to set reminders and control her home environment. By making these changes, Sarah was able to conserve energy and reduce the physical strain of daily tasks, allowing her to better manage her symptoms.

Another important adaptation is to **implement gentle exercise and stretching routines** tailored to your abilities. Regular physical activity, even in small amounts, can improve overall function and reduce pain. Activities like yoga, tai chi, or swimming are often beneficial as they promote flexibility and strength without putting excessive strain on the body. Always listen to your body and adjust the intensity of the exercise based on how you feel.

Finally, **mental and emotional adjustments** are also vital in adapting daily life. Accepting the need for rest and self-care without guilt is crucial. This might mean saying no to certain activities or delegating tasks to others. Building a support system of family, friends, and healthcare professionals who understand and support your needs can make a significant difference. Engaging in activities that bring joy and relaxation, such as reading, listening to music, or practicing mindfulness, can also help in maintaining a positive outlook.

Adapting daily life with fibromyalgia is about making thoughtful changes that allow you to live more comfortably and sustainably. By simplifying routines, using assistive tools, pacing activities, and incorporating gentle exercise, you can create a more manageable and fulfilling daily experience.

TIME AND ENERGY MANAGEMENT TECHNIQUES

Effectively managing time and energy is crucial for those living with fibromyalgia. The unpredictable nature of the condition means that what works one day may not be feasible the next. Developing adaptable strategies can help maintain productivity while conserving energy.

Prioritization and Planning: Start by listing daily tasks and categorizing them by priority. Focus on essential activities first, and break larger tasks into smaller, manageable steps. For instance, instead of cleaning the entire house in one go, tackle one room at a time over several days. This approach helps prevent overwhelming fatigue and ensures that critical tasks are completed.

Using a Planner: A planner can be an invaluable tool for managing your day. Record not only your tasks but also your symptoms and energy levels. This helps identify patterns and plan activities during peak energy times. For example, if you notice that mornings are when you feel most energetic, schedule demanding tasks for then, and leave more straightforward tasks for later in the day.

Pacing: Pacing involves balancing activity and rest to avoid overexertion. The "Spoon Theory," popularized by Christine Miserandino, is a helpful metaphor: imagine you have a limited number of spoons (units of energy) each day. Every task, no matter how small, uses up spoons. By being mindful of your "spoons," you can distribute your energy more effectively. For instance, if cooking a meal requires three spoons and you only have five for the day, plan accordingly to ensure you have enough energy left for other essential tasks.

Incorporating Breaks: Frequent breaks are essential to prevent burnout. For example, set a timer to remind you to rest for five to ten minutes every hour. During these breaks, engage in relaxing activities such as deep breathing, stretching, or listening to calming music. These short pauses can rejuvenate you, making it easier to tackle the next task.

Delegating Tasks: Don't hesitate to ask for help. Delegate tasks to family members or friends when possible. If budget allows, consider hiring professional help for chores like cleaning or yard work. Delegating not only reduces your workload but also conserves your energy for tasks that require your personal attention.

Technology Aids: Utilize technology to streamline tasks. Voice-activated assistants can help set reminders, make lists, or control home appliances, reducing the physical effort required. Apps for task management and symptom tracking can also help keep you organized and aware of your limits.

Flexible Scheduling: Flexibility is key in managing fibromyalgia. Some days will be better than others, and it's important to adjust your schedule accordingly. If you wake up feeling particularly fatigued, it's okay to reschedule non-essential tasks. This flexibility helps you listen to your body and respond to its needs without feeling guilty.

Mindfulness and Relaxation Techniques: Incorporating awareness-based exercises into your everyday schedule can greatly enhance your ability to regulate energy levels. Methods like focused breathing, systematic muscle easing, and visualized relaxation can alleviate tension and foster calmness, enabling you to better handle daily challenges. As an example, dedicating a brief period to conscious reflection can help clear mental clutter and reinvigorate your stamina, allowing you to tackle responsibilities with renewed focus and vigor.

Healthy Lifestyle Choices: Maintaining a balanced diet and staying hydrated can also play a role in managing energy levels. Eating small, frequent meals that include a mix of protein, healthy fats, and complex carbohydrates can prevent energy dips. Staying hydrated helps maintain overall energy and cognitive function. Regular, gentle exercise, as tolerated, can improve stamina and reduce pain over time.

Real-Life Example: Consider Jane, who has lived with fibromyalgia for five years. She uses a combination of pacing, prioritization, and delegation to manage her days. By keeping a detailed planner, she schedules demanding tasks when her energy is highest and includes regular breaks. Jane also practices mindfulness and relies on her family for support with household chores. This holistic approach allows her to maintain a productive lifestyle while managing her symptoms effectively.

Managing time and energy with fibromyalgia requires a multifaceted approach, including planning, pacing, and flexibility. By incorporating these techniques, you can create a more balanced and manageable daily routine, ultimately enhancing your quality of life.

CONCLUSION PART IV: LIVING WITH FIBROMYALGIA

Effective daily management strategies are a cornerstone of living well with fibromyalgia. By focusing on planning and organization, individuals can prioritize their tasks and manage their time more efficiently. Adapting daily life through small modifications can significantly reduce physical strain and enhance comfort. Furthermore, mastering time and energy management techniques helps maintain a balance between activity and rest, preventing burnout and promoting overall well-being.

The stories and examples provided in this chapter illustrate the resilience and creativity of individuals living with fibromyalgia. Their experiences highlight the importance of flexibility and adaptability in managing this condition. By incorporating these strategies into your daily routine, you can better navigate the challenges of fibromyalgia and improve your quality of life.

Remember, the journey to effective management is personal and unique. What works for one person may not work for another, so it's important to tailor these strategies to your specific needs and circumstances. By doing so, you can find a balance that allows you to live a fulfilling and productive life, even with fibromyalgia.

CONCLUSION

FINAL THOUGHTS AND ENCOURAGEMENT

As we wrap up this comprehensive guide on managing fibromyalgia, it's vital to acknowledge the journey you've undertaken. Living with fibromyalgia is not merely a medical challenge; it's a daily testament to your resilience, adaptability, and strength. Every day you push forward, you demonstrate an incredible amount of courage. This book was designed to be more than just a resource; it's a companion, a source of support and guidance through your toughest times.

Recognize Your Achievements: It's easy to overlook the progress you've made, especially when symptoms can fluctuate so unpredictably. Take a moment to appreciate the small victories. Maybe today you managed to get out of bed a little earlier, or you found a meal plan that works for you. These achievements, no matter how small they may seem, are steps toward a better quality of life. Celebrating them can fuel your motivation and provide a sense of accomplishment.

Build and Rely on Your Support Network: Having a strong support system is crucial. Whether it's friends, family, or support groups, surrounding yourself with people who understand and empathize with your condition can make a significant difference. Don't hesitate to lean on them. Their support can provide emotional relief and practical help, making daily management easier. Sharing your experiences and hearing theirs can also offer new perspectives and strategies you might not have considered.

Practice Self-Compassion: On tough days, it's crucial to be gentle with yourself. Fibromyalgia can be relentless, and it's natural to feel overwhelmed. Allow yourself to rest when needed and engage in activities that bring you joy and relaxation. Practicing mindfulness and meditation can help center your thoughts and reduce stress. Remember, self-care is not a luxury but a necessity for managing your condition effectively.

Stay Informed and Open-Minded: The landscape of fibromyalgia research and treatment is constantly evolving. Stay informed about new developments, but also be discerning. Not every new treatment or strategy will work for everyone. It's important to listen to your body and work closely with your healthcare providers to find what suits you best. Being proactive about your health is empowering and can lead to discovering new ways to alleviate your symptoms.

Advocate for Yourself: Navigating the healthcare system can be daunting, but being your own advocate is essential. Communicate openly with your doctors about your symptoms, treatment preferences, and any concerns you have. Don't be afraid to seek second opinions or explore new therapies. Your voice matters, and ensuring your healthcare providers understand your experiences can lead to better, more personalized care.

Hold onto Hope: Living with fibromyalgia can sometimes feel like an uphill battle, but hope is a powerful ally. Advances in research and treatments continue to emerge, offering new possibilities for relief and improved quality of life. Stay hopeful and proactive, seeking out information and resources that can support you in your journey.

This book is here to remind you that you are not alone. Each page is filled with strategies, tips, and stories to guide you through your daily challenges. Remember, your journey with fibromyalgia is unique, and your strength, resilience, and determination will carry you through. Keep pushing forward, and know that better days are ahead. You have the tools, the knowledge, and the support to live a fulfilling life, despite the challenges fibromyalgia presents.

CONTINUING YOUR HEALING JOURNEY

The path to managing fibromyalgia is ongoing, and it is essential to view it as a dynamic process rather than a destination. Embracing this perspective can transform how you cope with daily challenges and help you remain open to new possibilities for relief and improvement.

First, let's talk about adaptability. The symptoms of fibromyalgia can fluctuate, sometimes unpredictably. One day you might feel relatively okay, and the next day, the pain and fatigue could be overwhelming. This inconsistency can be frustrating, but cultivating adaptability in your approach can make a significant difference. If you wake up on a difficult day, consider modifying your plans instead of pushing through as usual. This might mean rescheduling activities or adjusting your workload. Flexibility allows you to respond to your body's needs more compassionately.

Second, continuous learning is crucial. The medical community is constantly researching fibromyalgia, leading to new insights and treatments. Stay informed about the latest developments by following reputable sources, engaging with fibromyalgia communities, and discussing new information with your healthcare providers. For example, if you read about a new dietary approach or a promising therapy, bring it up at your next medical appointment to see if it might be suitable for you.

Third, self-reflection plays a vital role. Regularly take time to reflect on what strategies are working and what might need adjustment. Keeping a journal can be a helpful tool for this. Document your symptoms, what you did that day, what you ate, and how you felt. Over time, patterns may emerge that can guide your management plan. For instance, you might discover that certain foods consistently trigger flares, or that specific activities help alleviate symptoms.

Fourth, seek and give support. Being part of a supportive community can significantly impact your journey. Engage with support groups, whether in person or online, to share experiences, tips, and encouragement. These interactions not only provide emotional support but can also offer practical advice from those who understand your struggles firsthand. Moreover, consider how you can support others. Sharing your experiences and what you've learned can be incredibly empowering and foster a sense of purpose and connection.

Fifth, prioritize mental and emotional well-being. Living with a chronic condition like fibromyalgia can take a toll on your mental health. It's vital to incorporate practices that support your emotional well-being. Mindfulness, meditation, and relaxation techniques can help manage stress and improve your overall outlook. If you're struggling, don't hesitate to seek professional help from a therapist or counselor who understands chronic pain conditions.

Sixth, celebrate your progress. It's easy to focus on setbacks, but acknowledging your achievements, no matter how small, is essential. Whether it's a day with less pain, successfully implementing a new coping strategy, or maintaining a positive mindset despite challenges, these are victories worth celebrating.

Finally, maintain hope and perseverance. Fibromyalgia can be daunting, but remember that you have the strength to navigate this journey. Advances in medical research and increased awareness continue to improve understanding and treatment of fibromyalgia. Stay hopeful and persistent in finding what works best for you. Every effort you make towards managing your condition contributes to a better quality of life.

Your journey with fibromyalgia is uniquely yours, and with the tools and knowledge you've gained, you are better equipped to handle its challenges. Keep moving forward with resilience, knowing that each step you take is a testament to your strength and determination.

ACKNOWLEDGEMENTS

Writing this book has been an intense and emotional adventure, and there are so many people I want to thank from the bottom of my heart.

First and foremost, a huge hug goes to my family.

Mom, your love and strength have been my beacon in the darkest moments. You've always listened to me during my outbursts, offering an understanding ear when I needed it most.   And you, my love, my companion in life, you've always understood and supported me. On days when my energy was low, you did the work of two, showing a dedication that goes beyond all expectations. And how could I forget you, my little ball of fur? Your sweet meows and purrs have been the best medicine in moments of pain.

A special thought goes to you, dear readers. I hope that these pages of my book have given you not only useful tools but also a glimmer of hope and the certainty that you're not alone in this battle. Your stories and your strength have inspired me every day, and I'm deeply grateful to be able to share this journey with you.

As a small token of appreciation for reading the book, I've prepared a special gift for you: the **FibroTracker: Your Personal Symptom and Pain Journal**. It's a special diary designed for fibromyalgia patients. It's not just a simple log, but a real tool to track symptoms and pain, providing a clear and detailed picture of your daily health status. This will help you better understand your body and manage your condition more effectively.

Always remember that even on the toughest days, you're not alone. There are always new paths to explore, new hopes to discover. Keep fighting, keep searching, keep hoping. You're incredibly strong and capable, never give up.

With all my love and gratitude,

Liv Marwin

To download your free
FIBROTRACKER
Your Personal Symptom & Pain Journal,

simply scan the QR code below.

SCAN ME

This tool is designed to help you track your symptoms,
medications, and overall progress each day.
Just print it out and fill it in as needed.

If you enjoyed this book and found it helpful,
I would greatly appreciate it
if you could share your thoughts.

Please scan the QR code below to leave your opinion.

Thank you for your support!

You can print the FibroTracker pages directly from the QR code, making it easy to have a physical copy on hand.
Alternatively, **FibroTracker Your Personal Symptom & Pain Journal** is available on <u>Amazon</u> if you prefer a professionally bound version.

FIBROTRACKER
Your Personal Fibromyalgia Chronic Pain & Symptom Tracker Journal A Detailed Daily Record to Monitor Symptoms, Triggers, and Medications - Empowering You to Control Your Fibromyalgia Journey

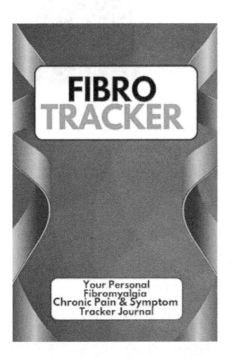

Made in the USA
Monee, IL
09 November 2024